This book belong to the strongest warrior:

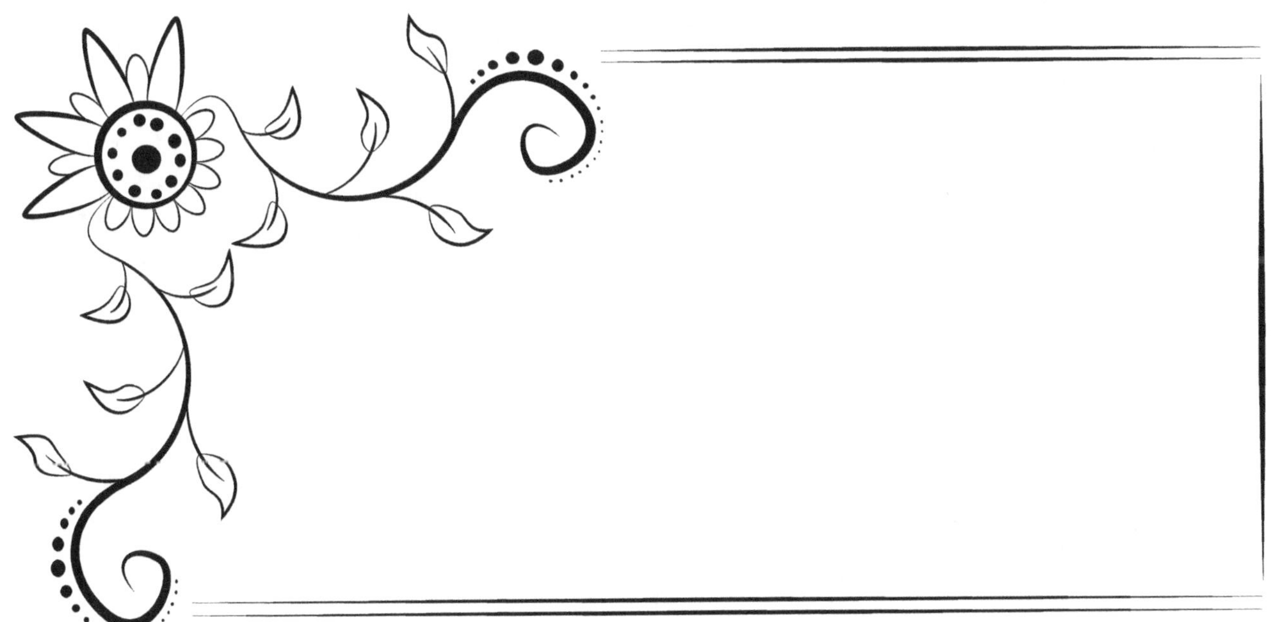

Colors Testing

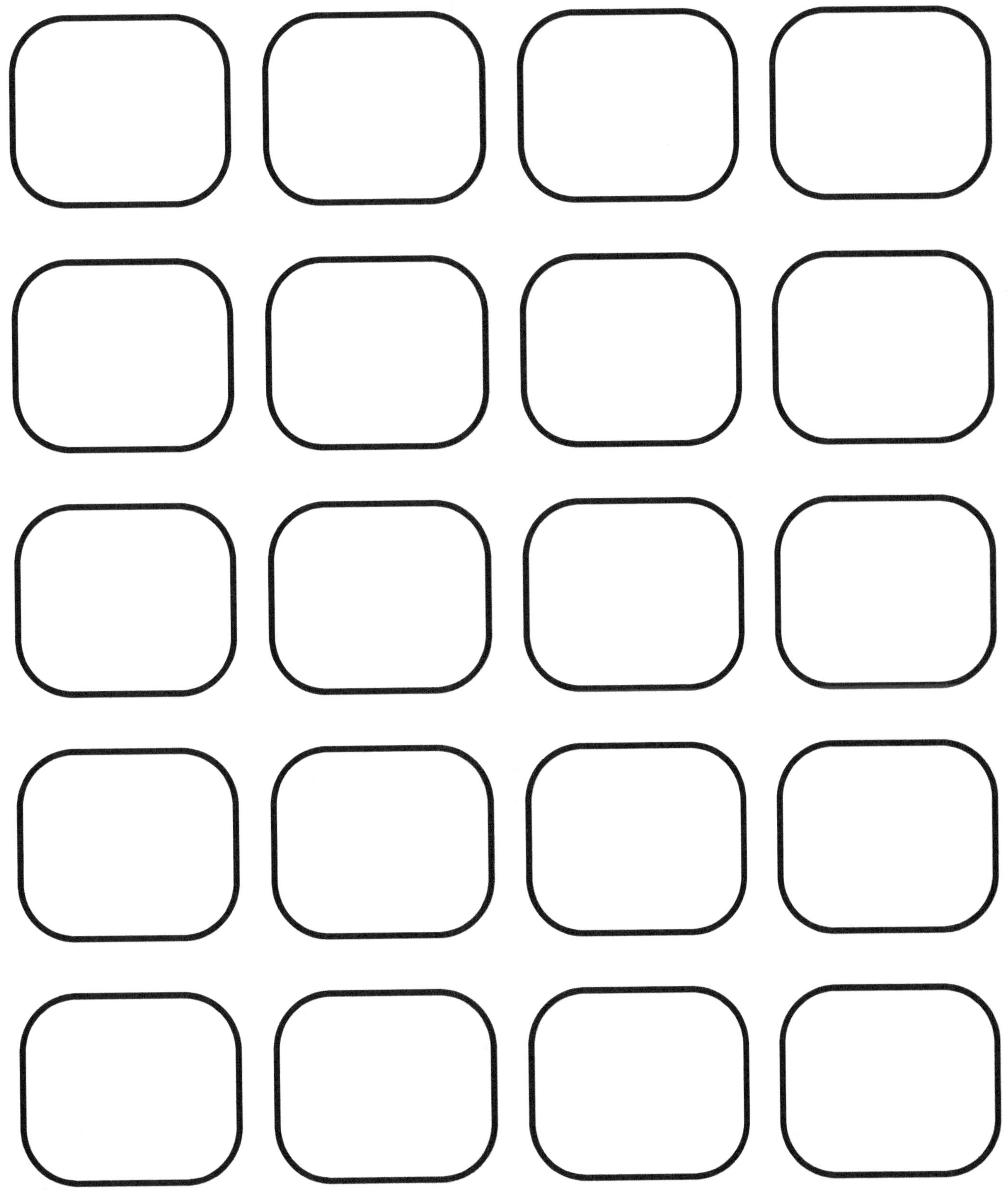

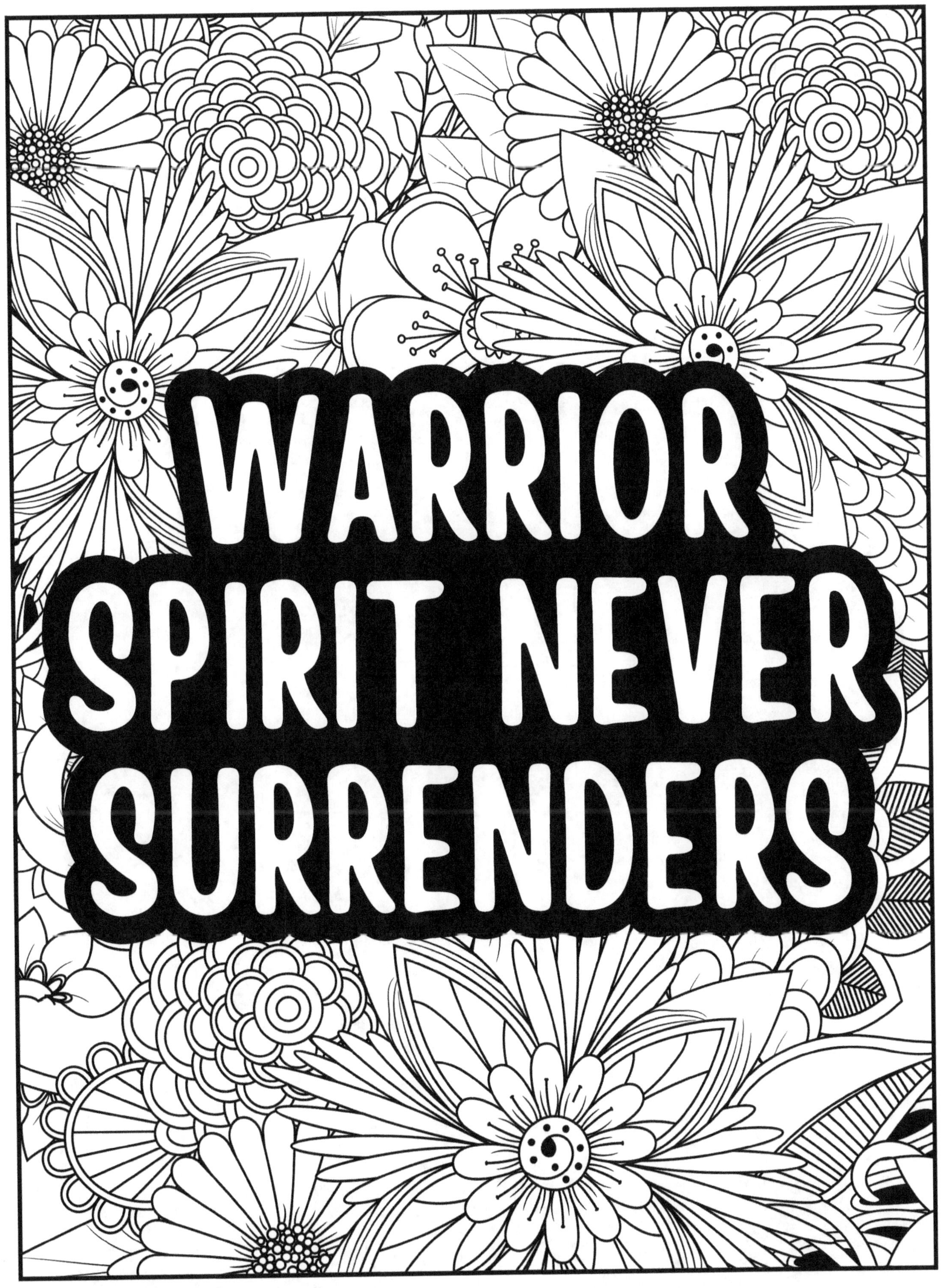

WARRIOR
SPIRIT NEVER
SURRENDERS

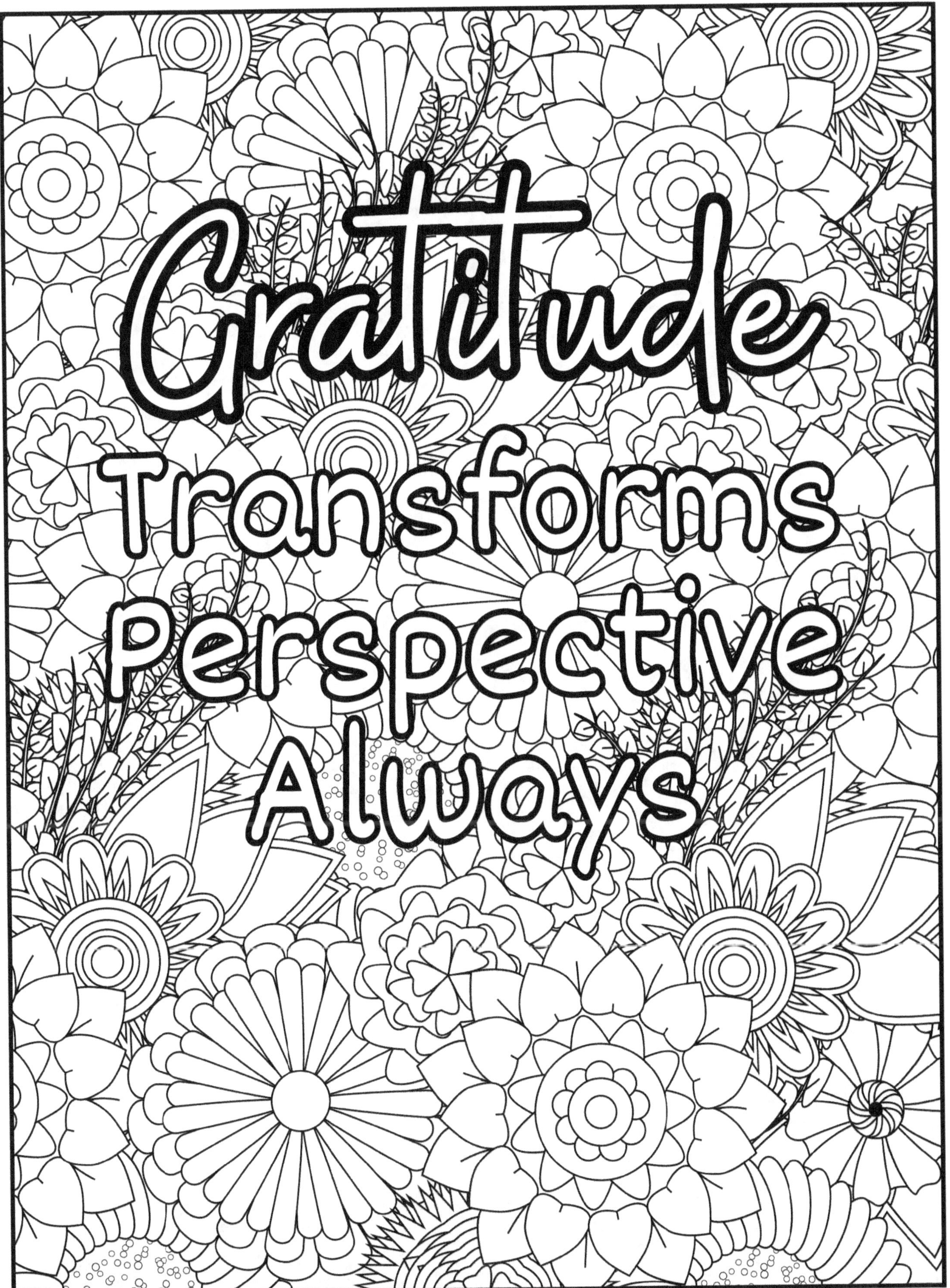
Gratitude
Transforms
Perspective
Always

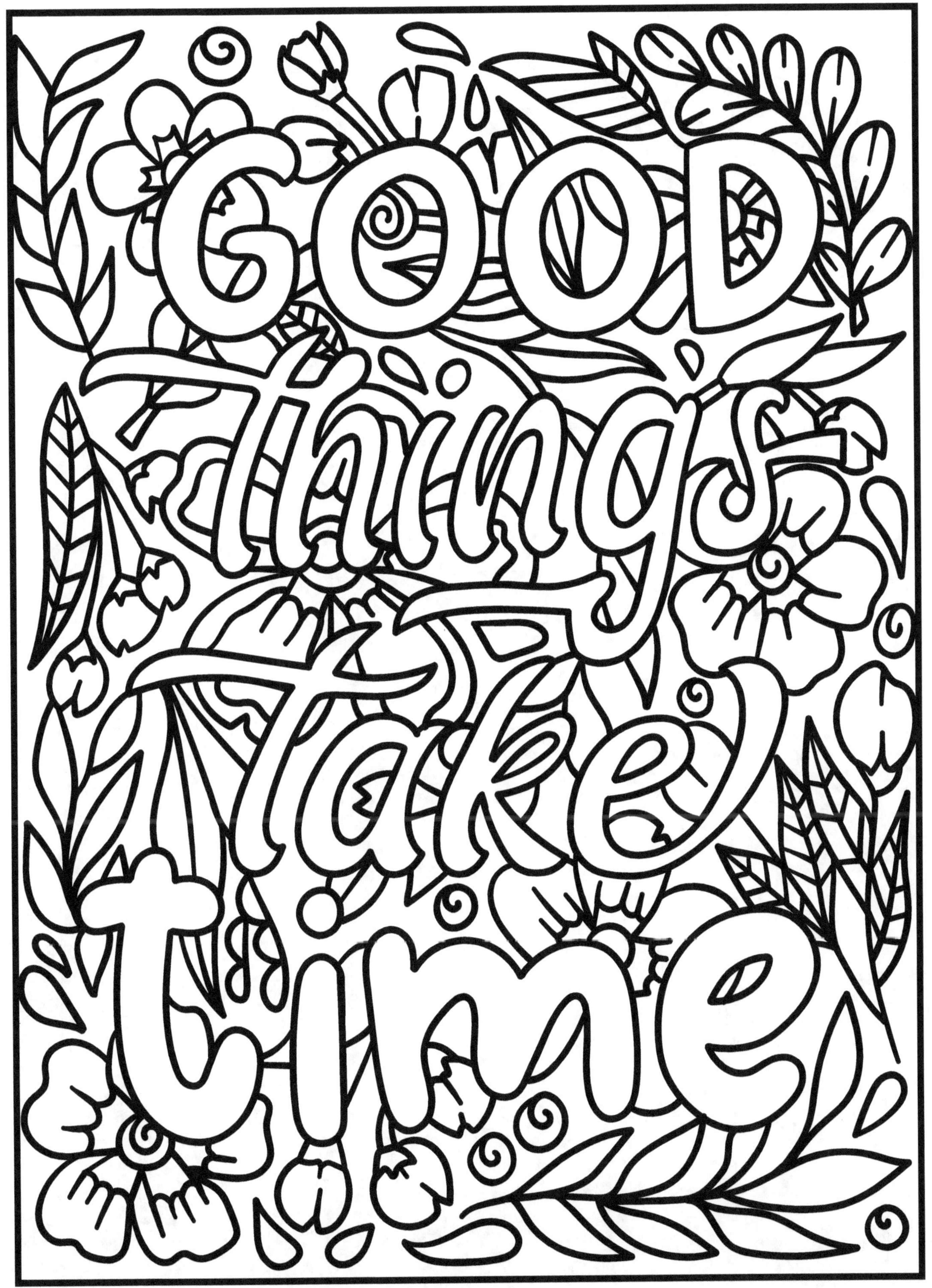

GOOD
things
take
time

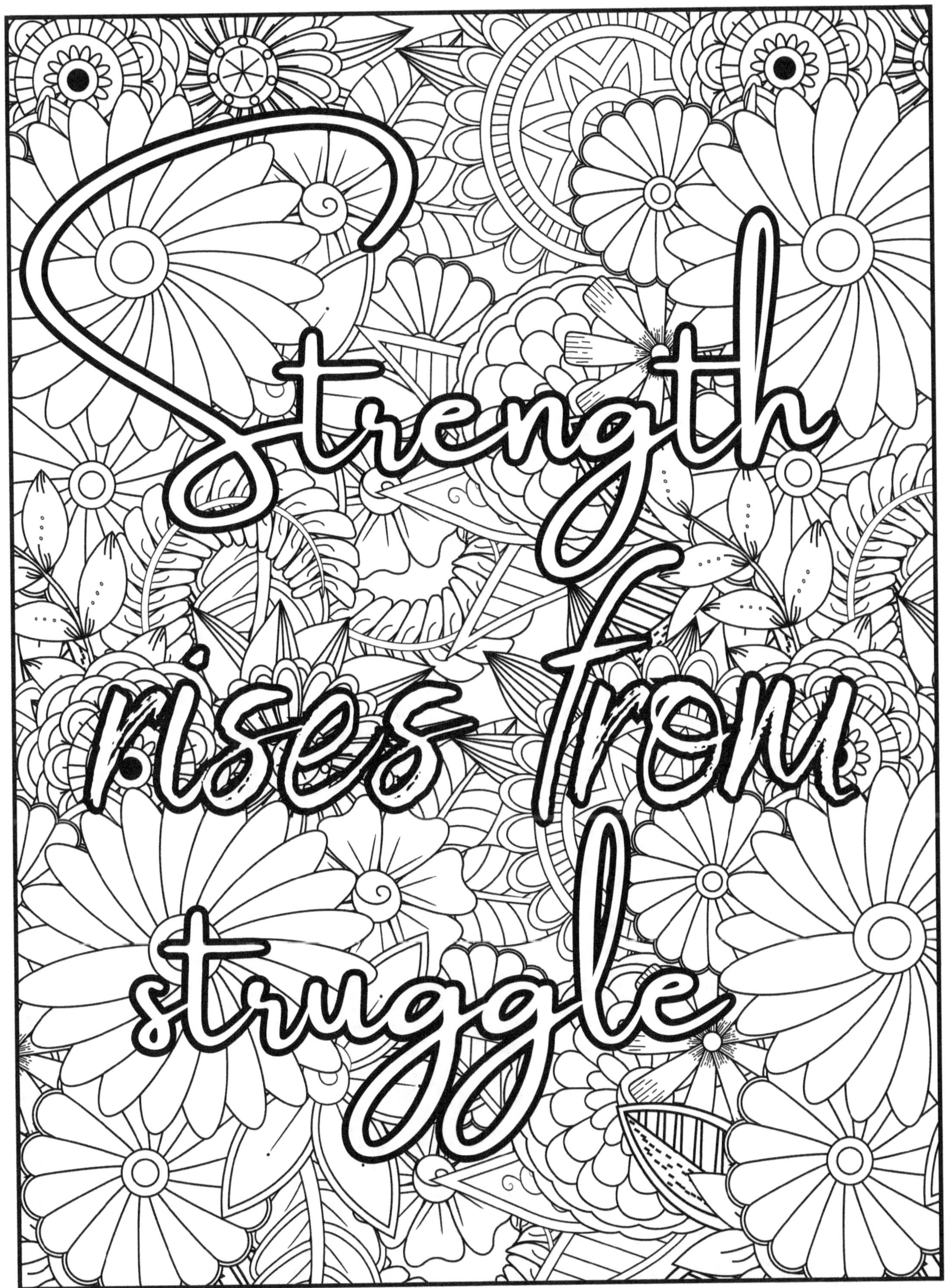

Strength
rises from
struggle

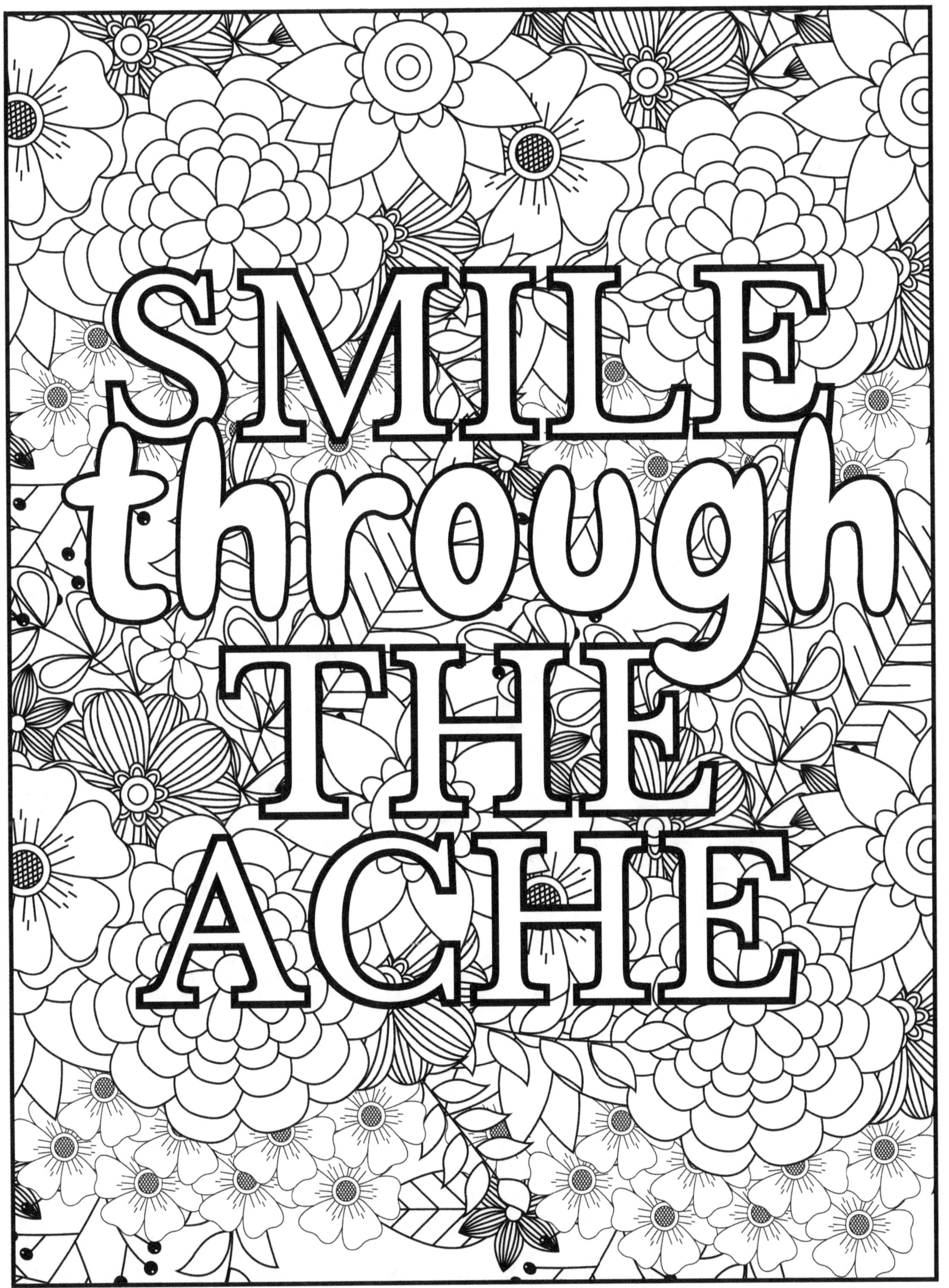

SMILE
through
THE
ACHE

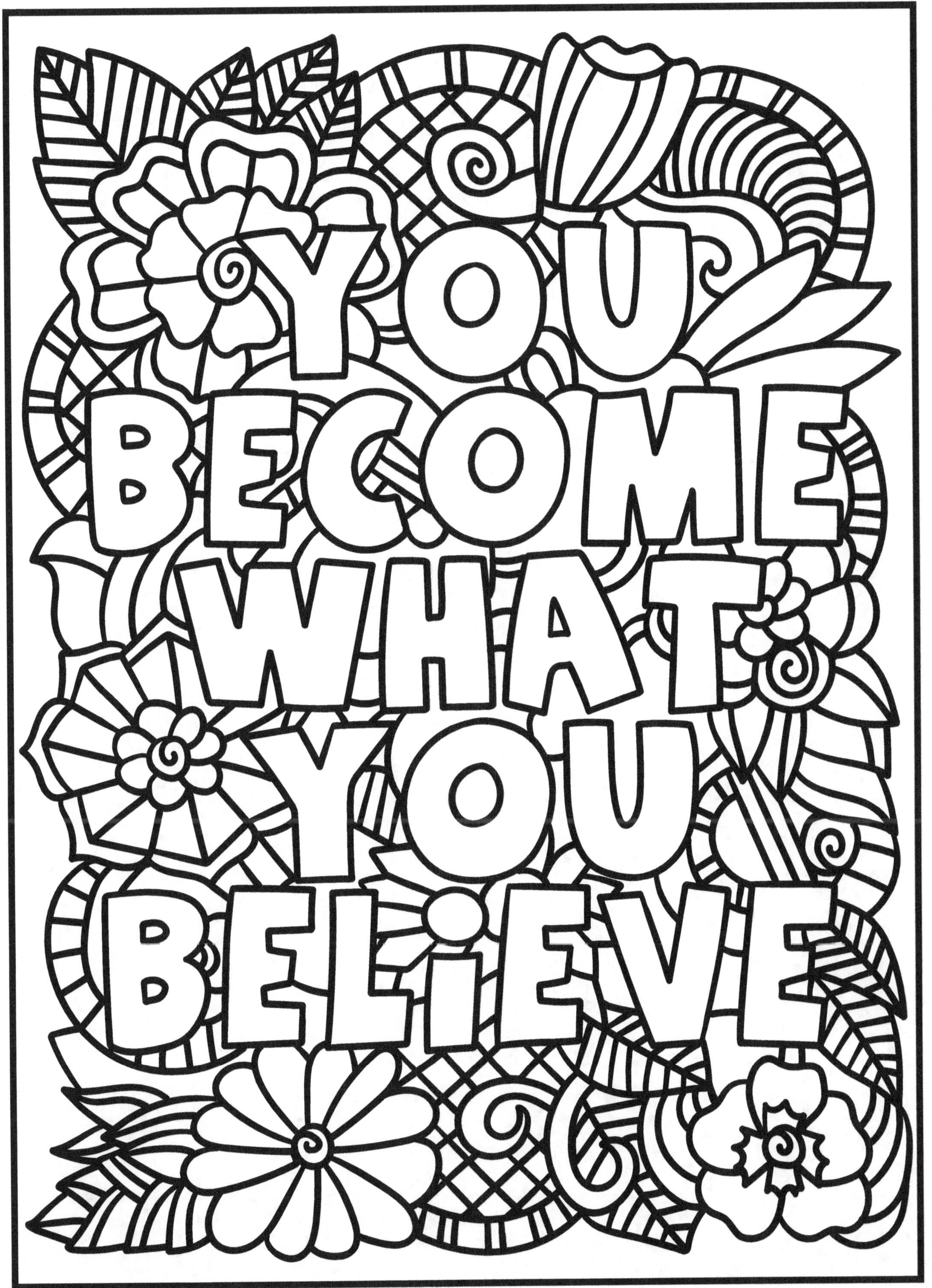

YOU
BECOME
WHAT
YOU
BELIEVE

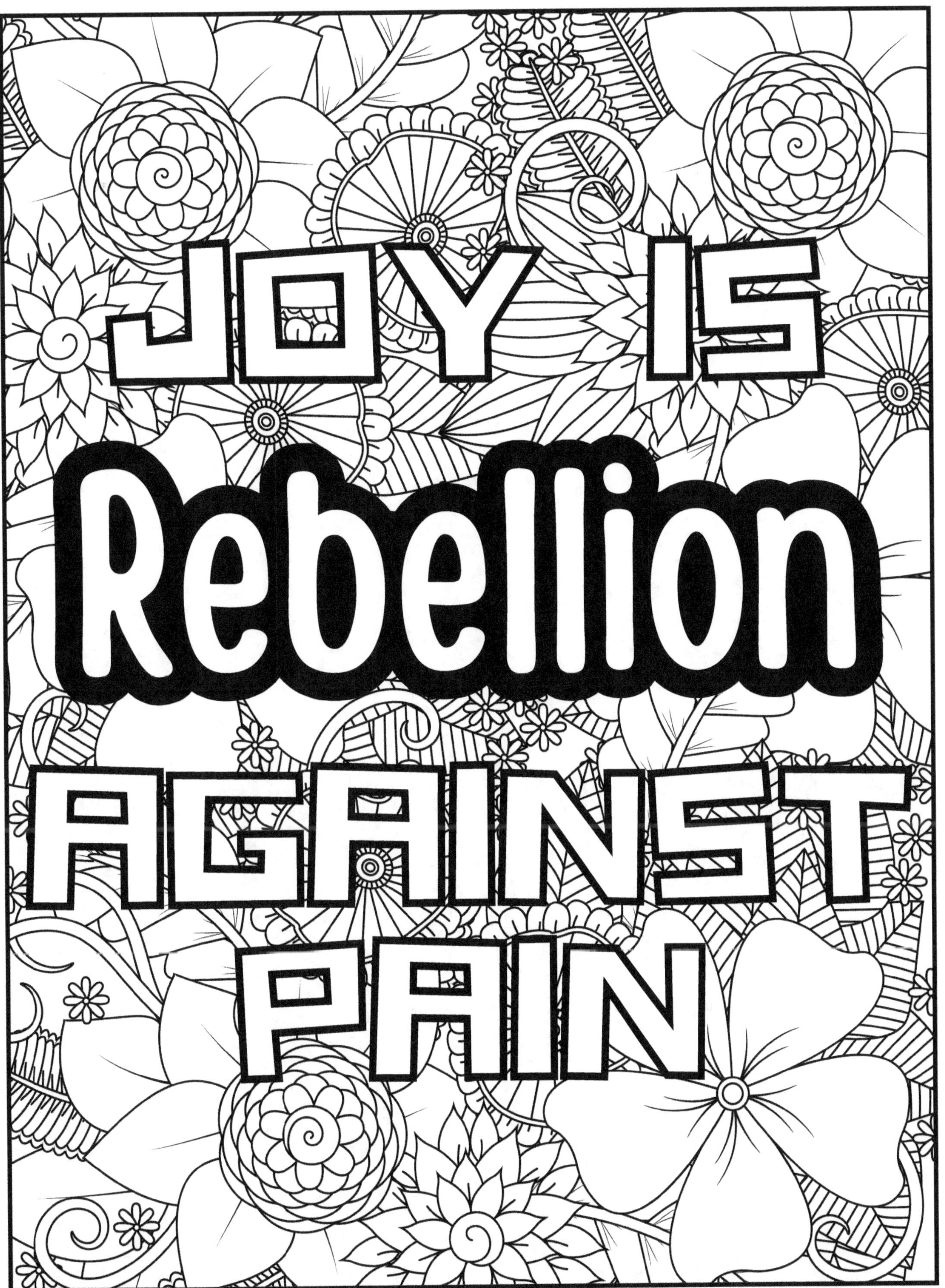

JOY IS
Rebellion
AGAINST
PAIN

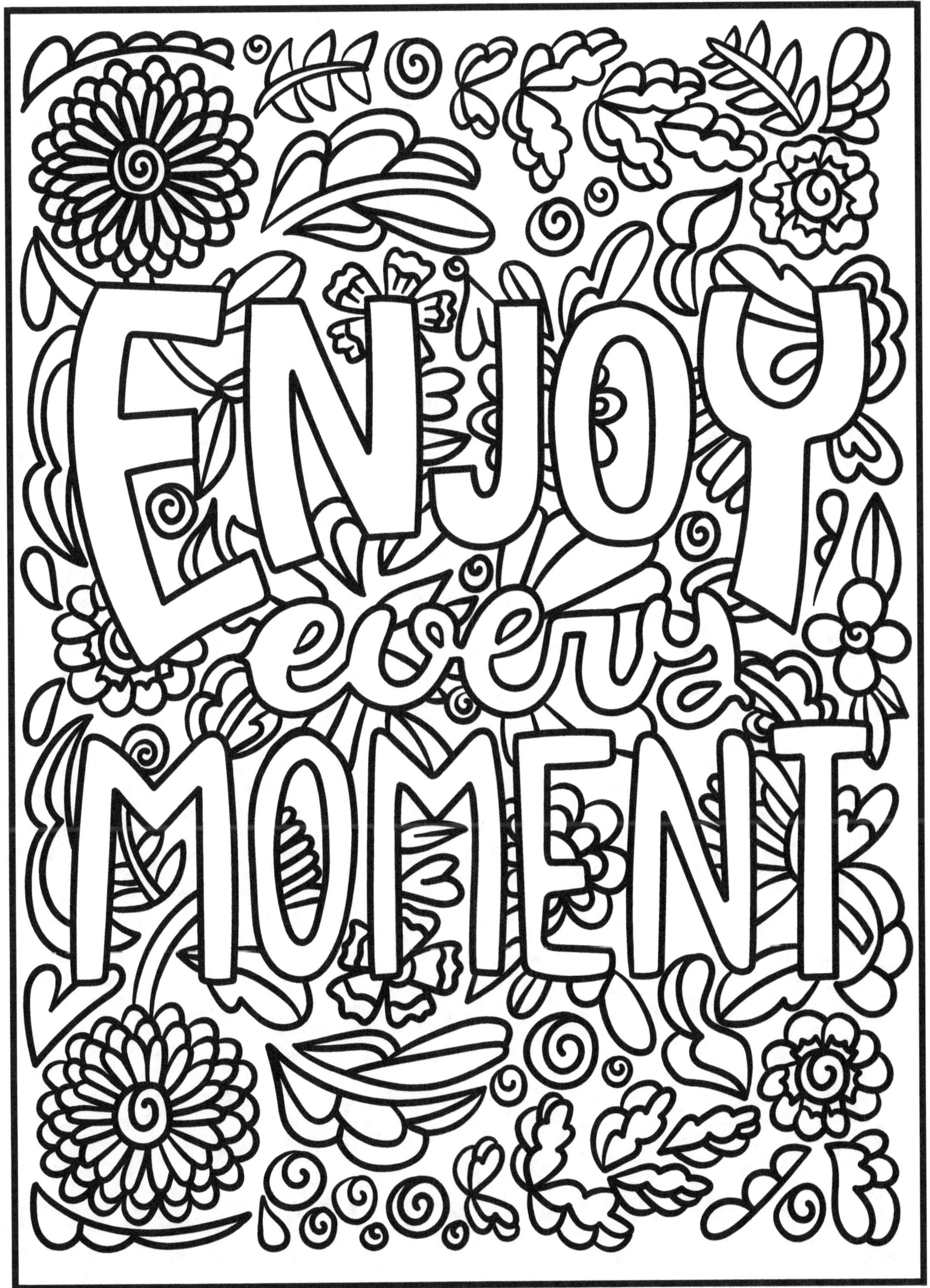

ENJOY
every
MOMENT

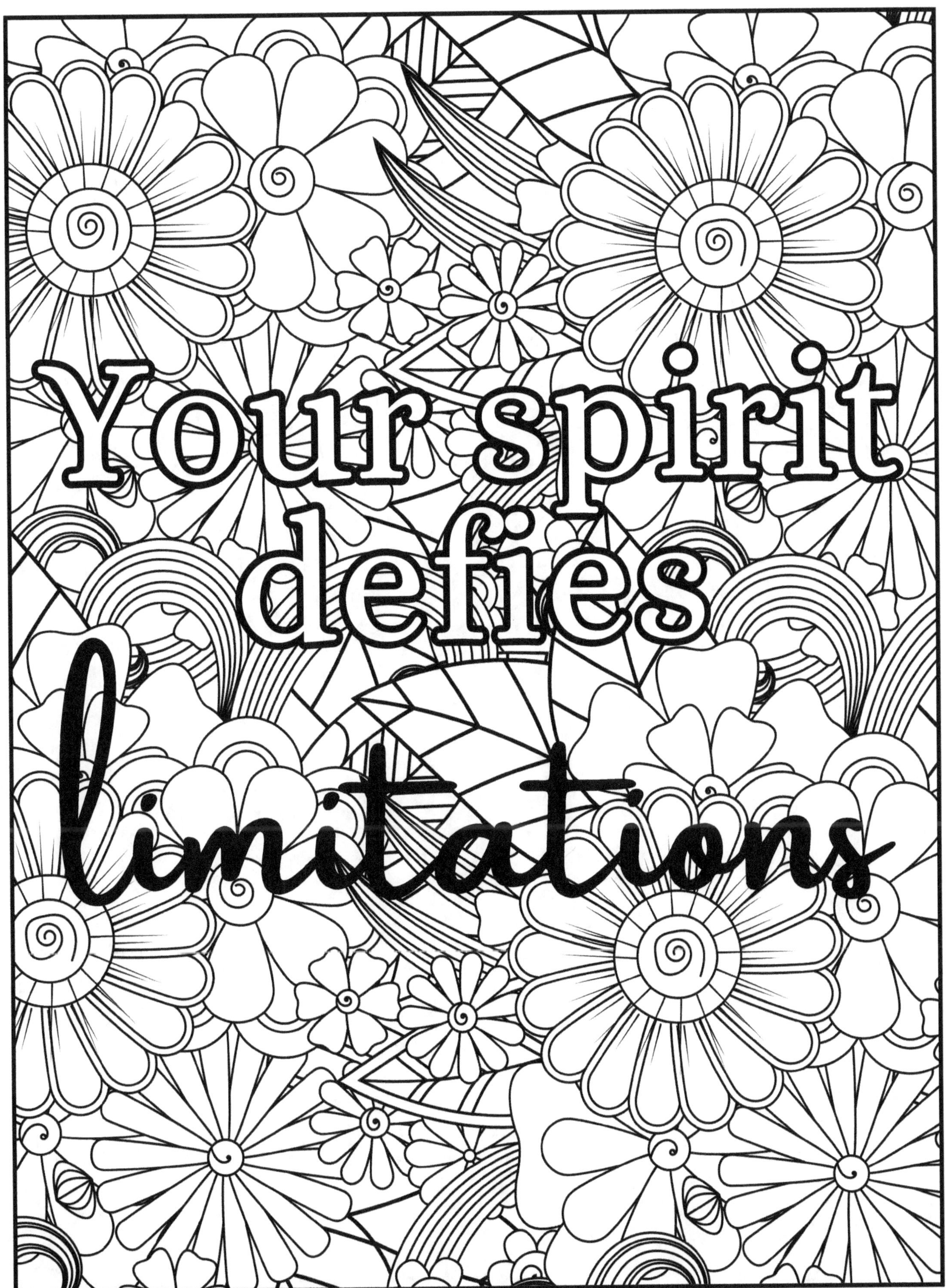

Your spirit
defies
limitations

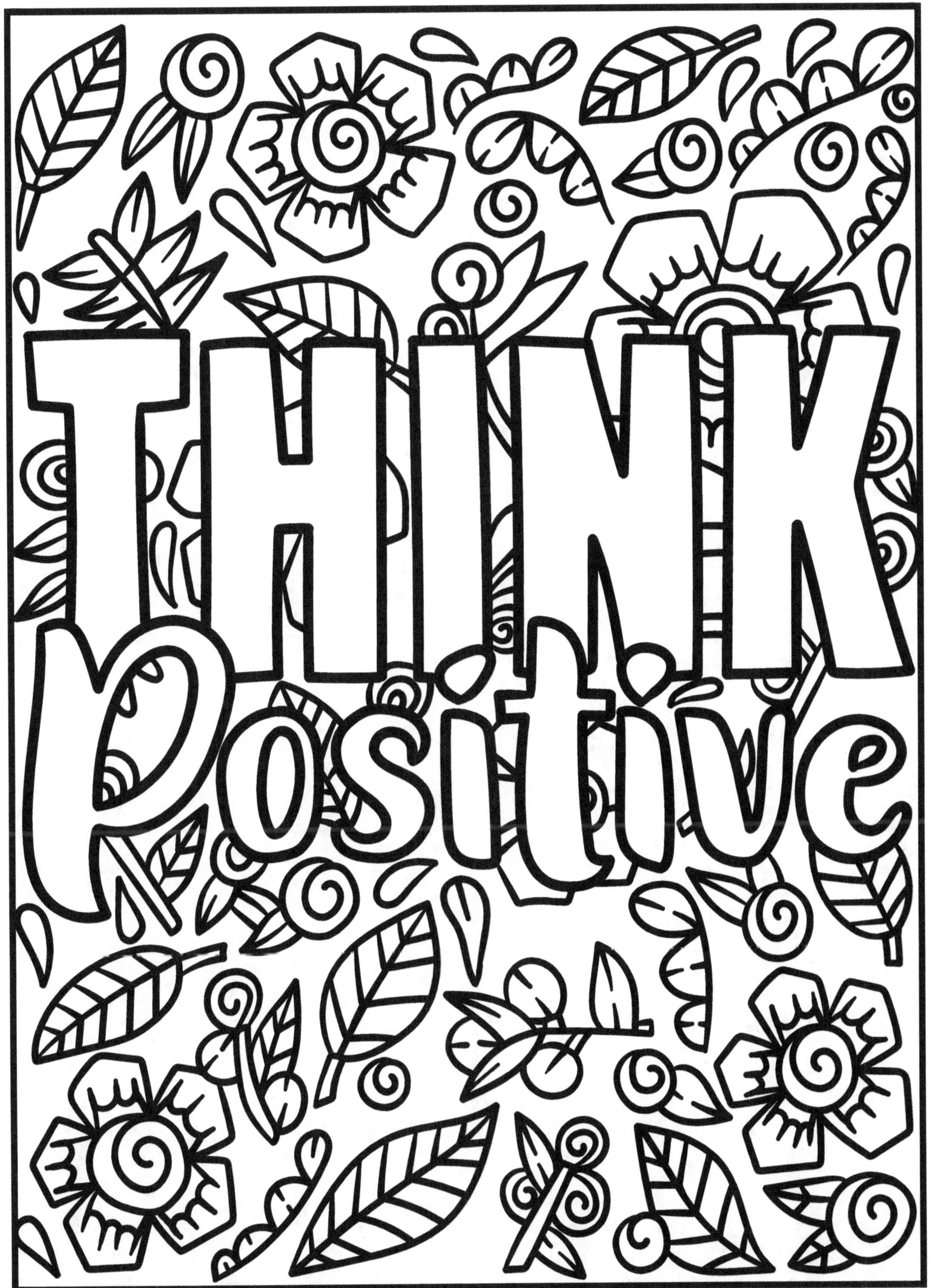
THINK
Positive

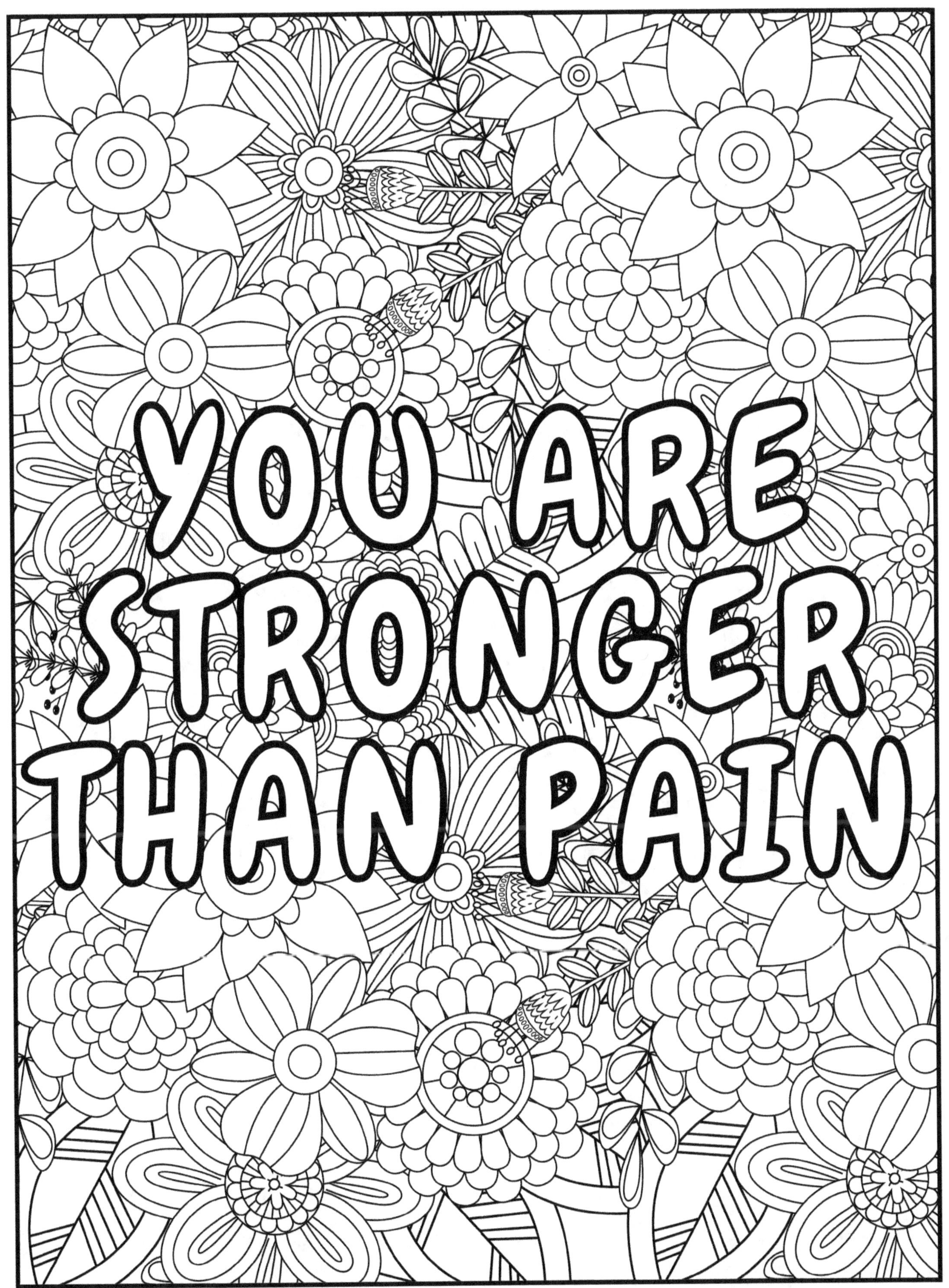

YOU ARE
STRONGER
THAN PAIN

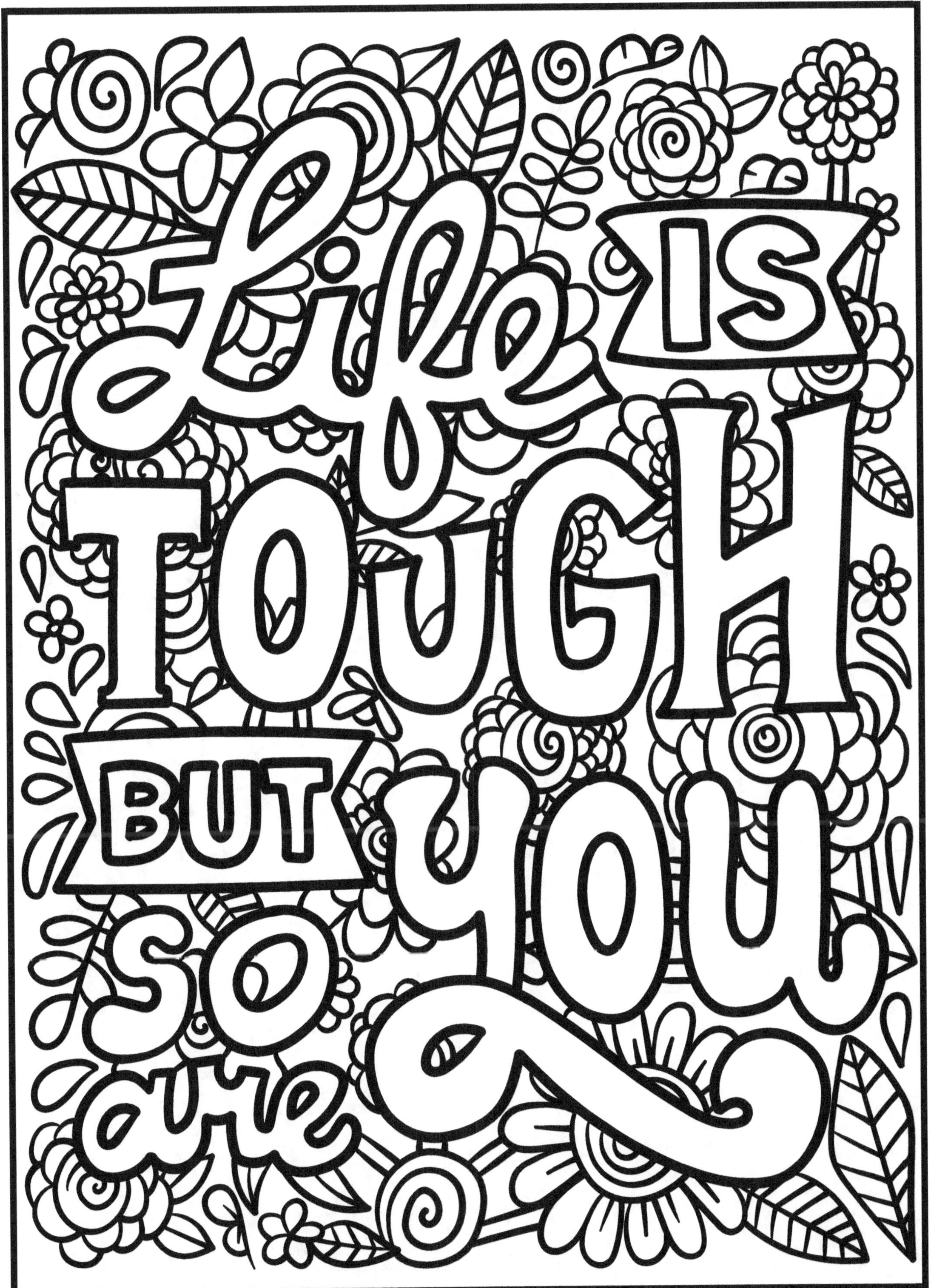

Life is
Tough
But So you
are

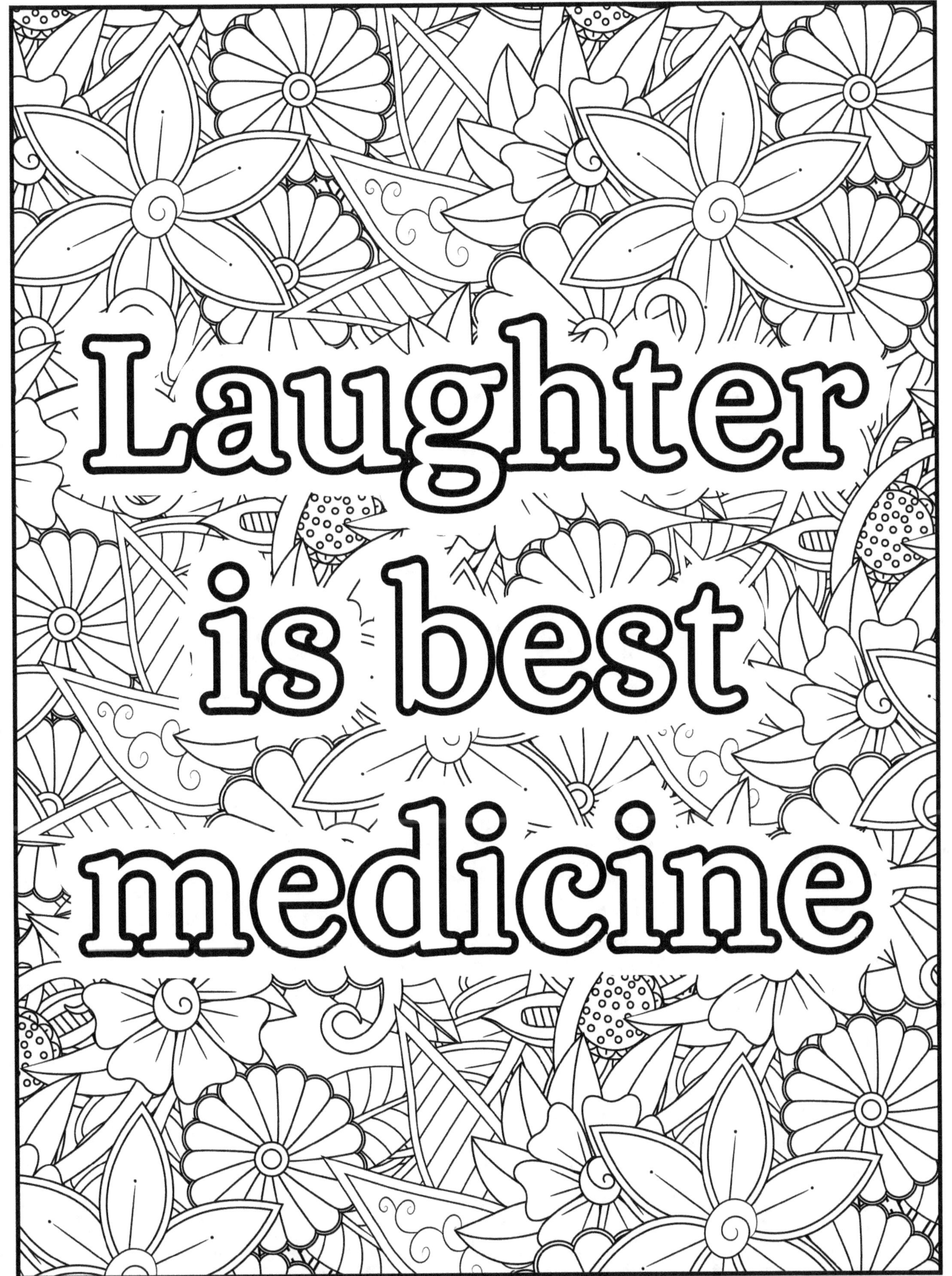
Laughter
is best
medicine

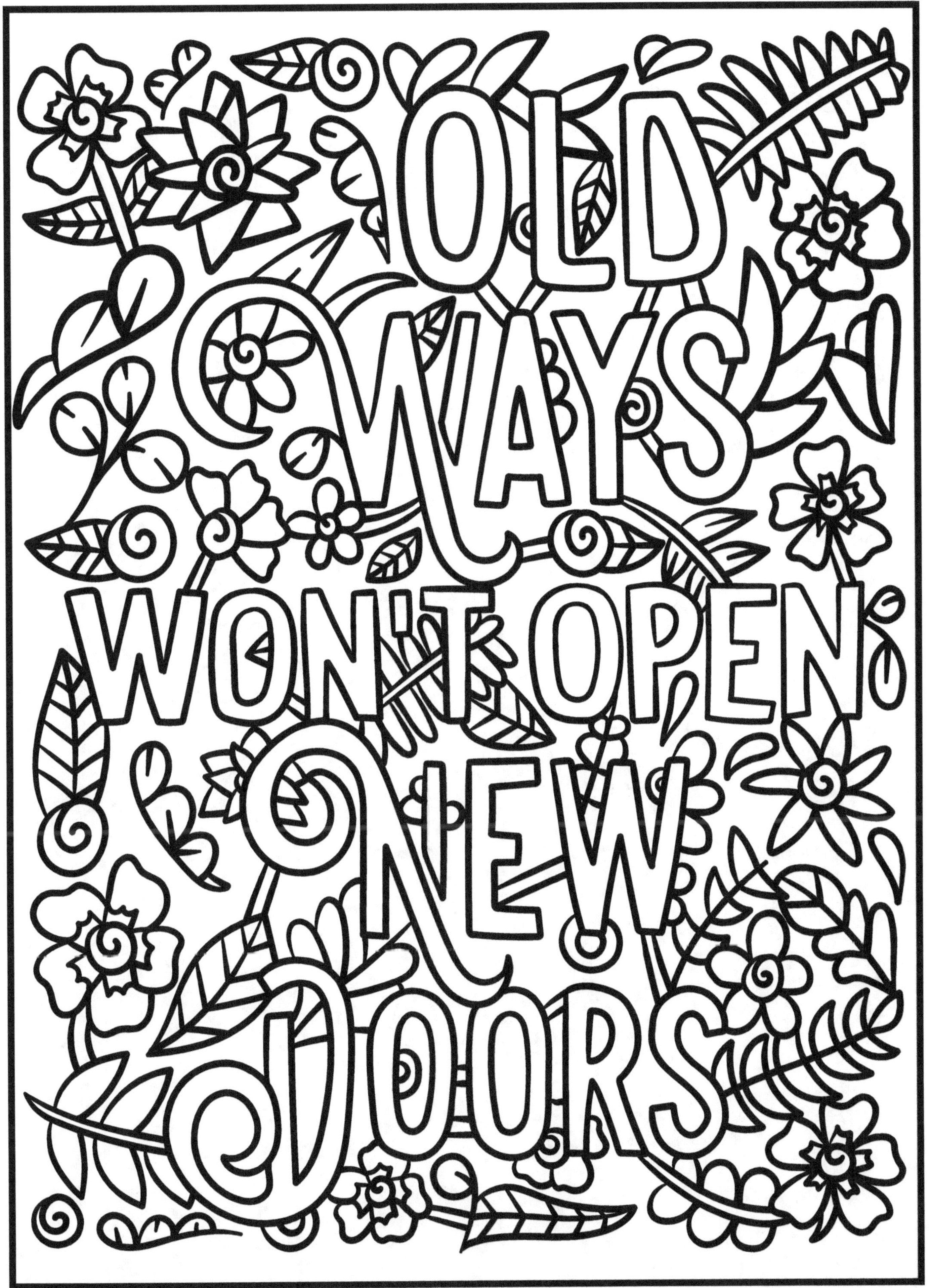

OLD
WAYS
WON'T OPEN
NEW
DOORS

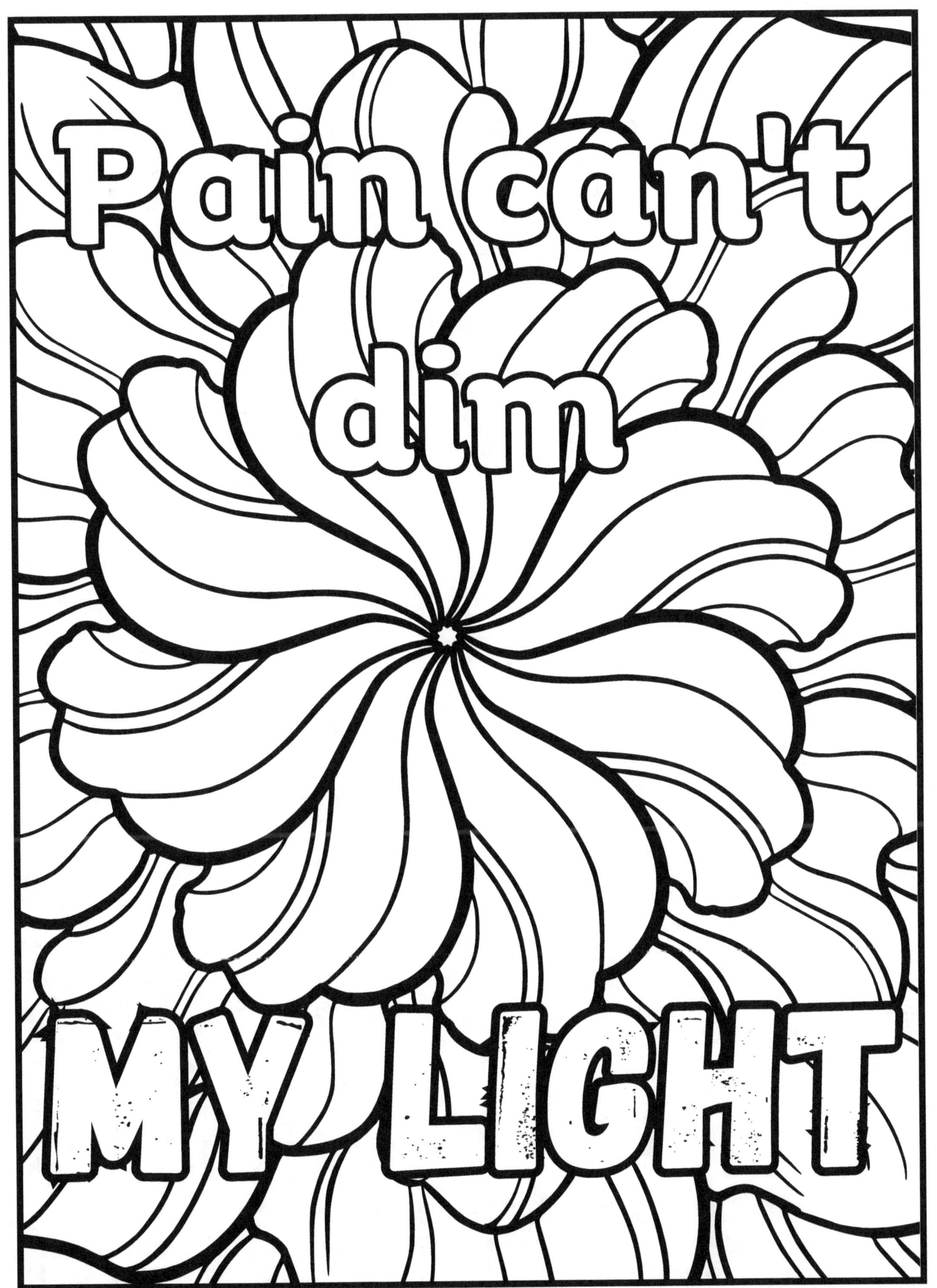

Pain can't dim
MY LIGHT

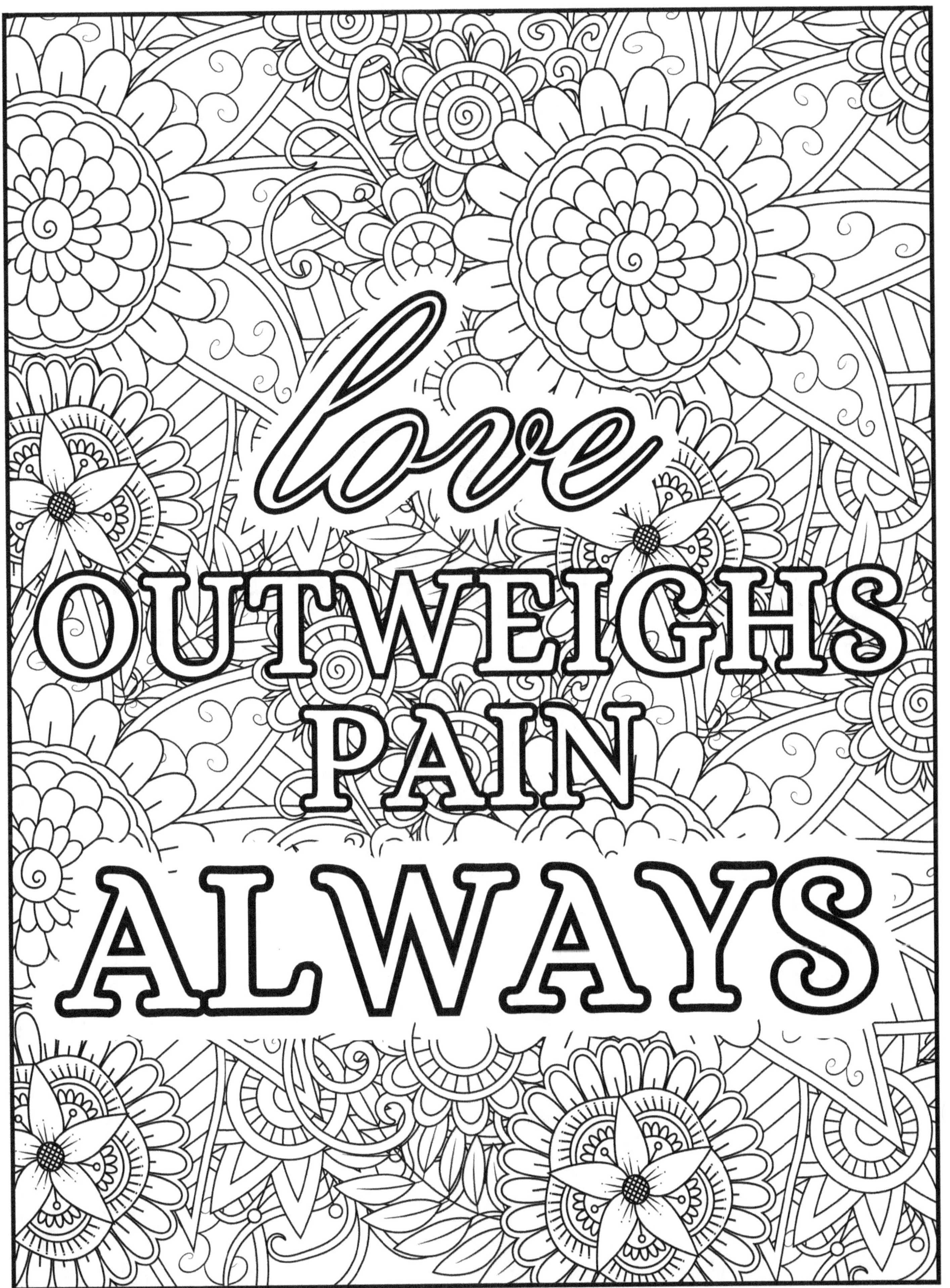

love
OUTWEIGHS
PAIN
ALWAYS

RAINBOWS

After Storms

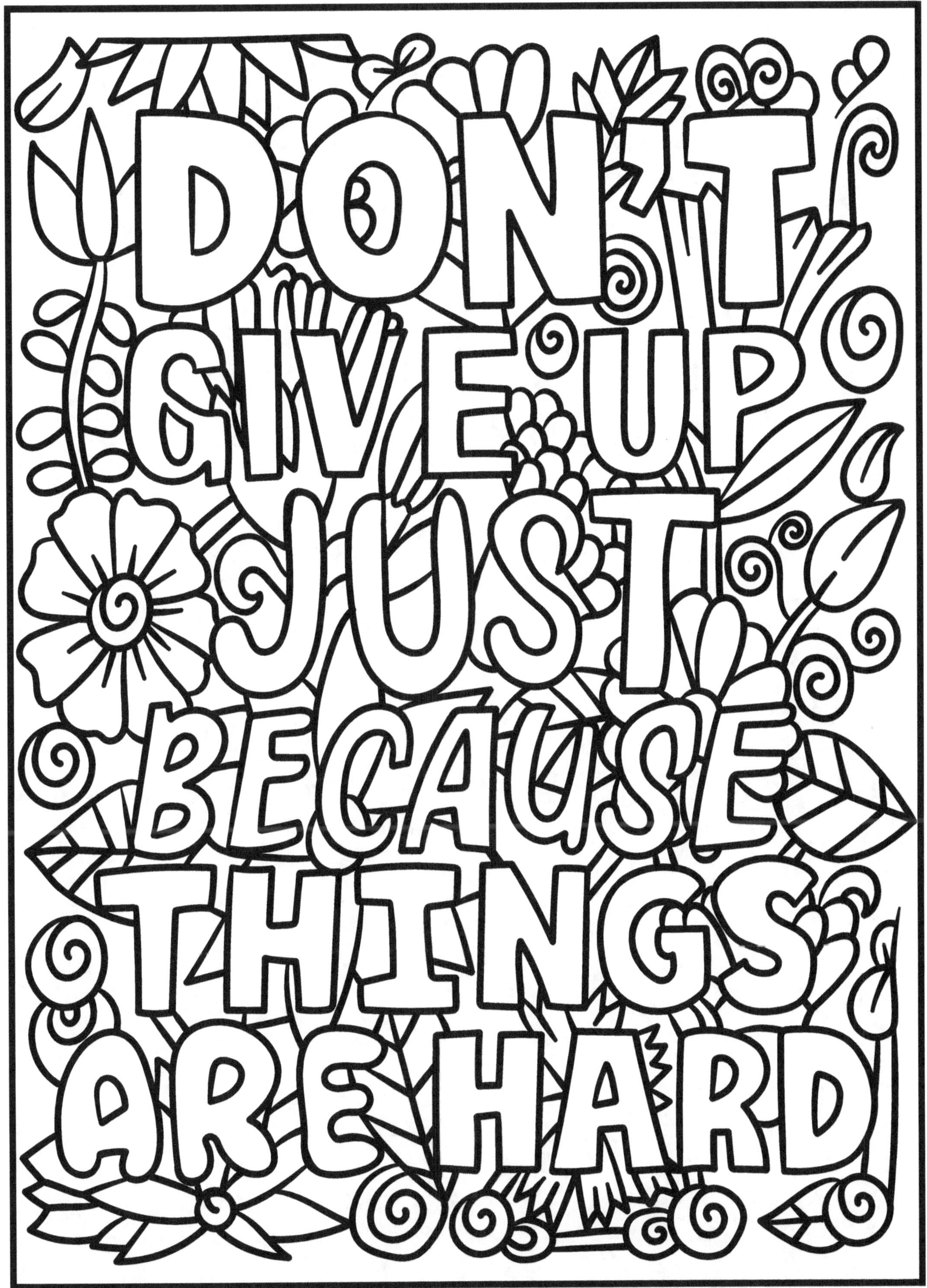

DON'T
GIVE UP
JUST
BECAUSE
THINGS
ARE HARD

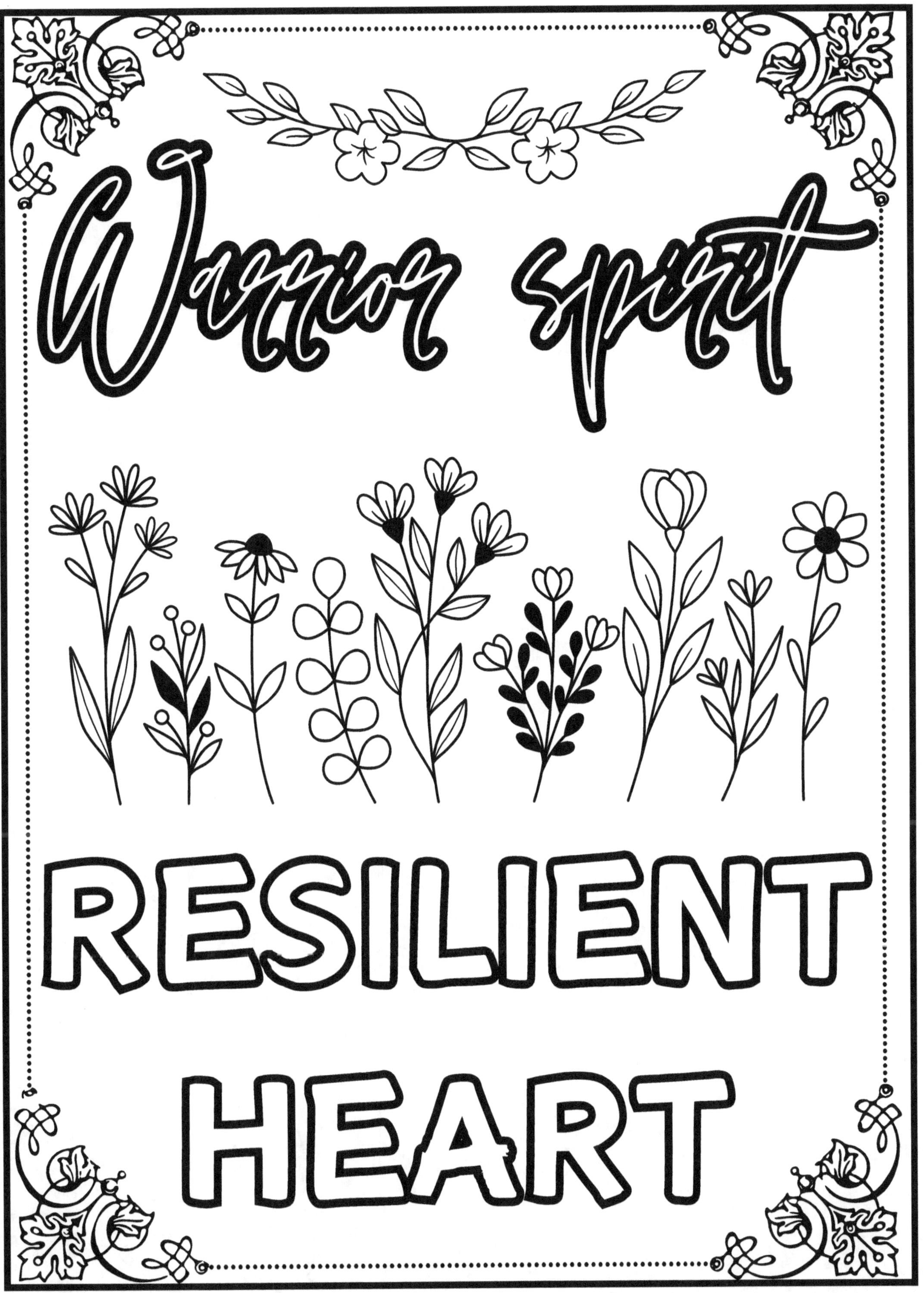

Warrior spirit
RESILIENT
HEART

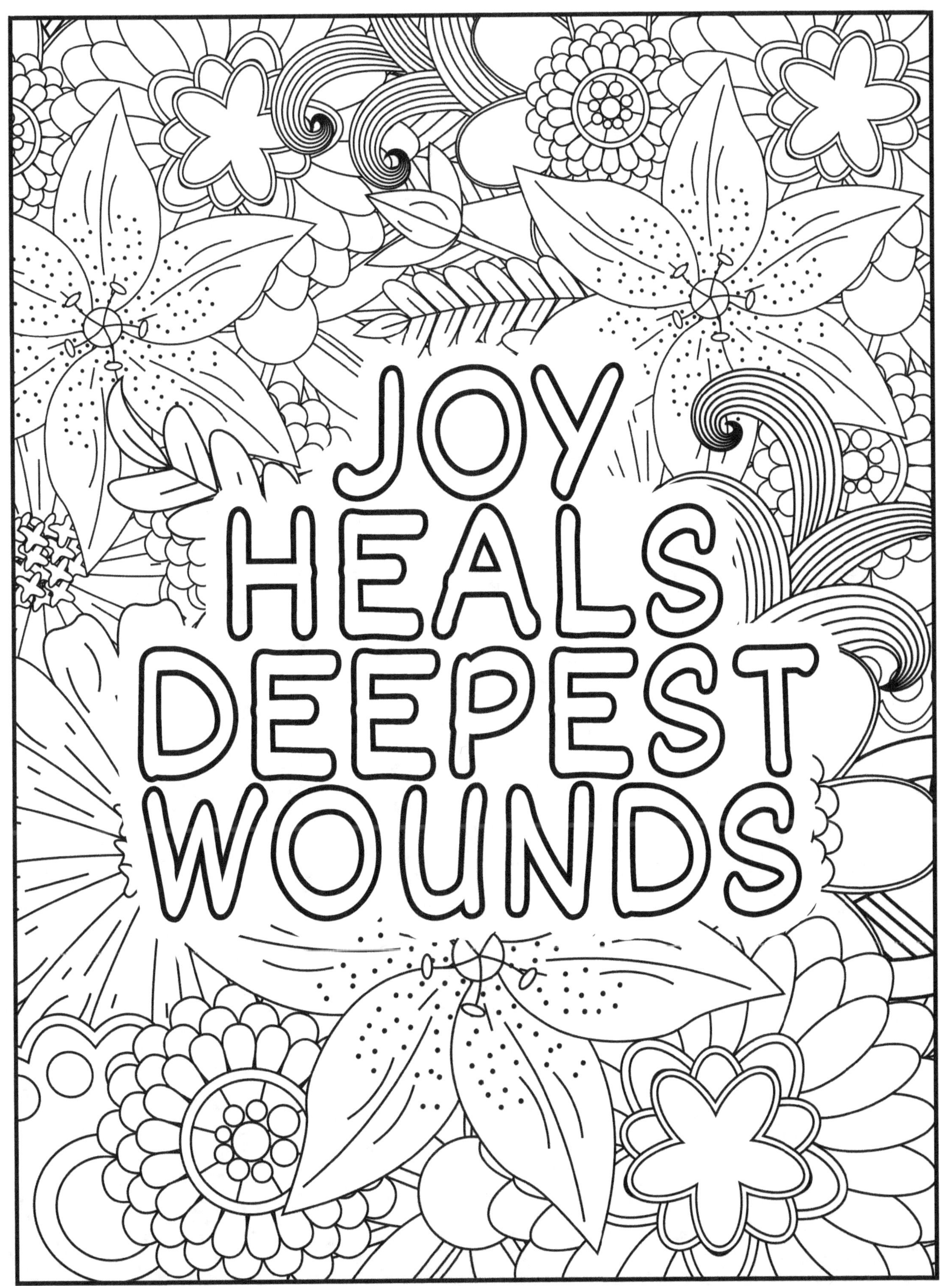

JOY
HEALS
DEEPEST
WOUNDS

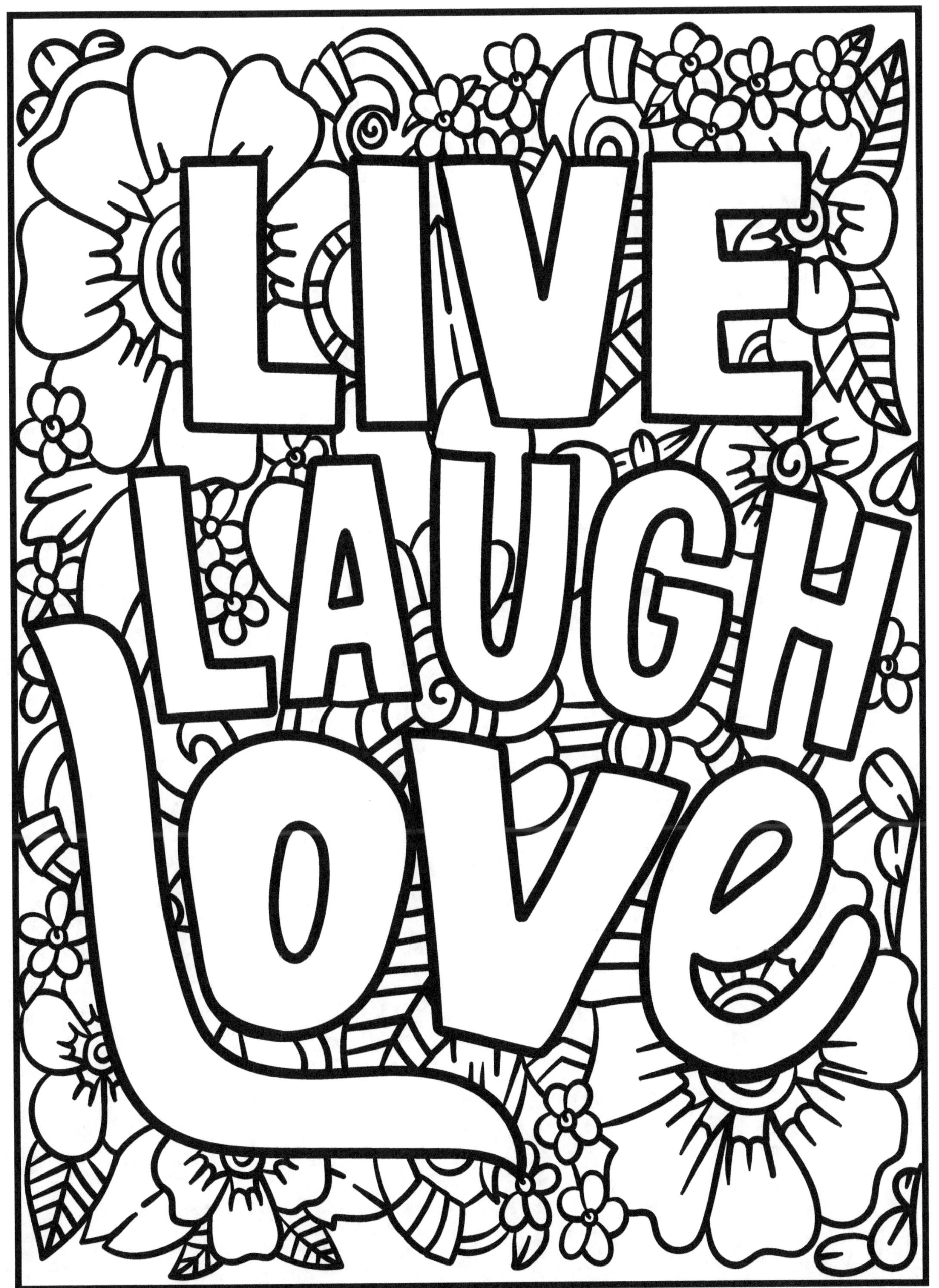
LIVE
LAUGH
love

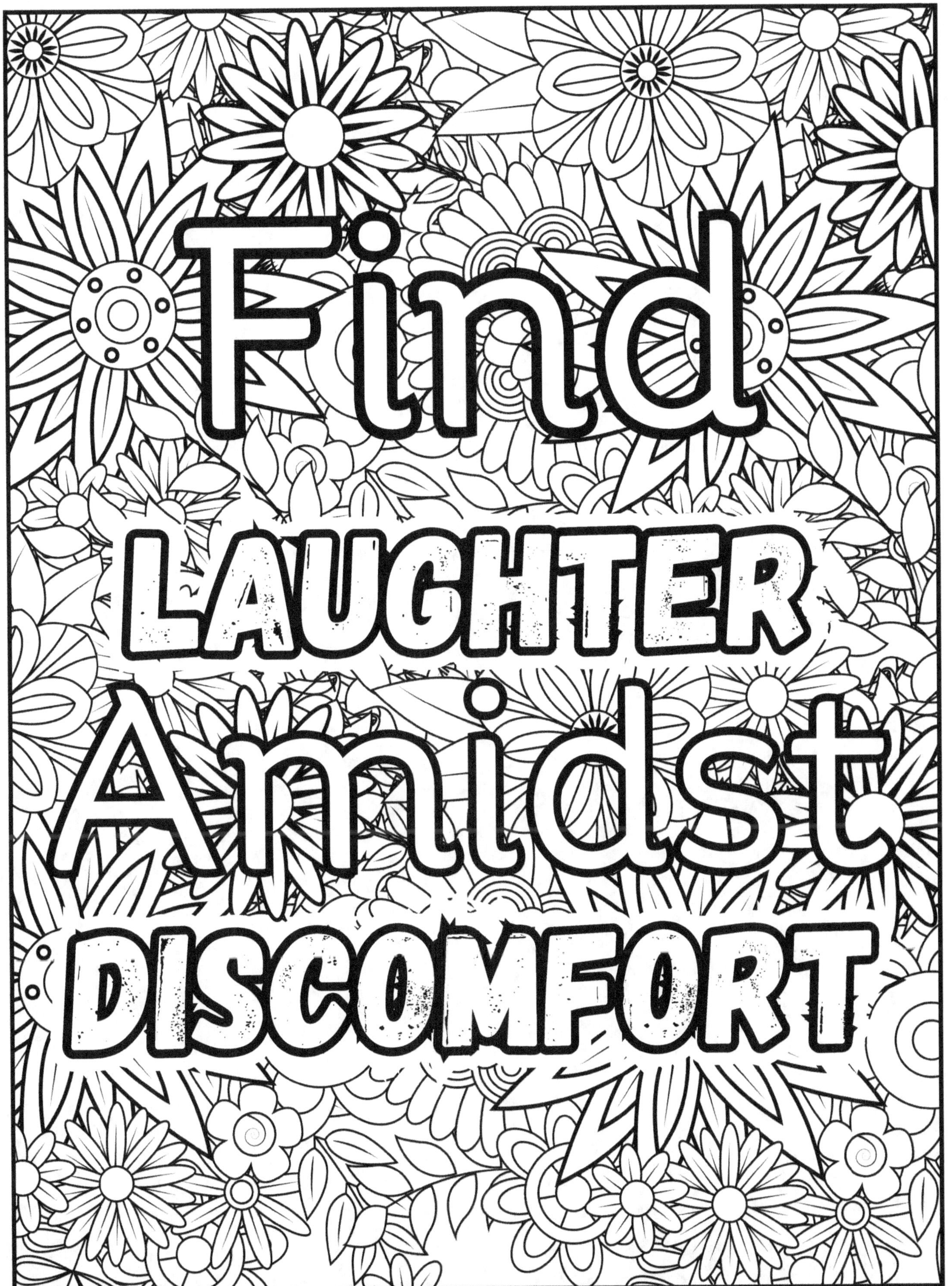

Find
LAUGHTER
Amidst
DISCOMFORT

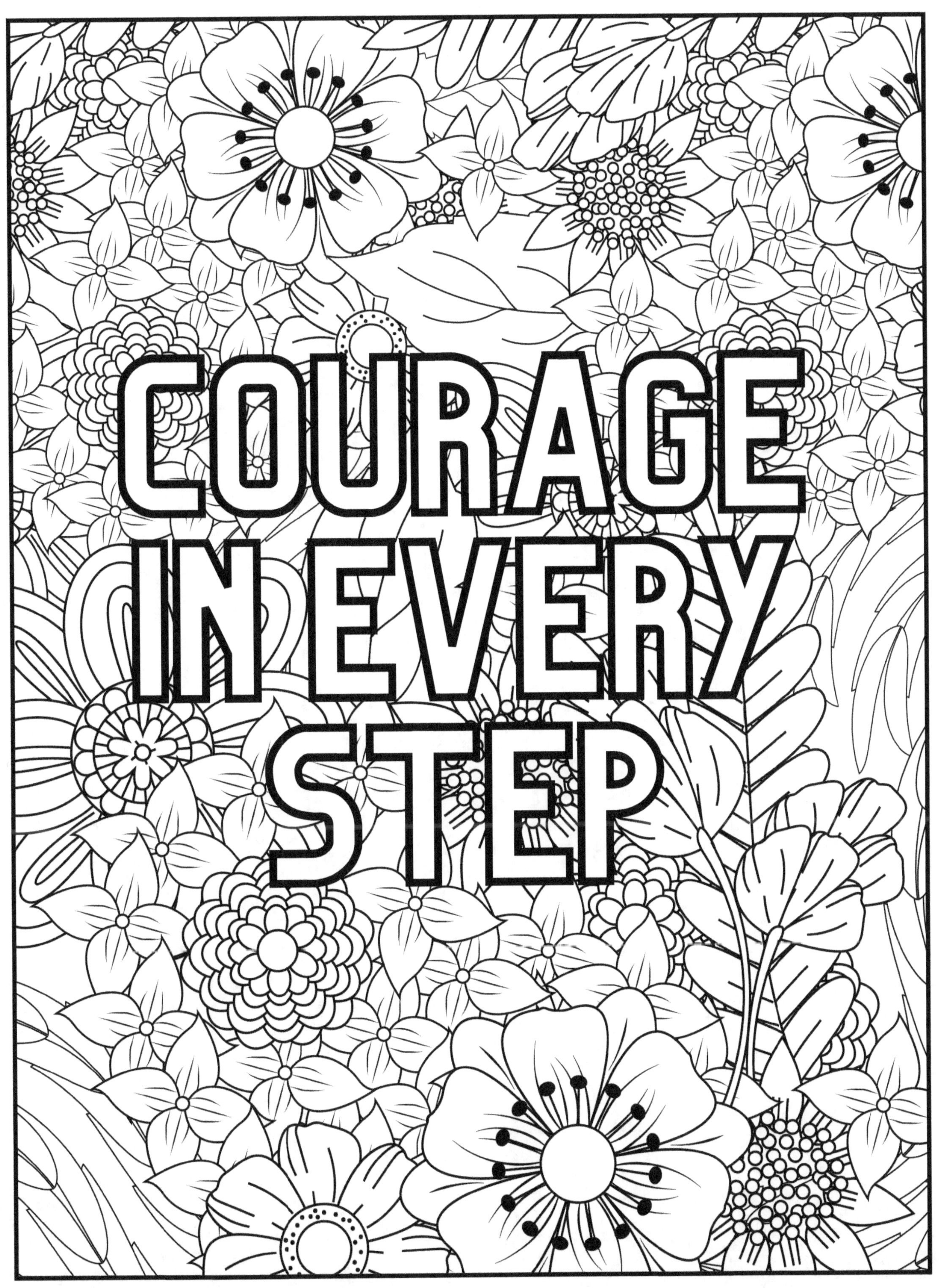

COURAGE
IN EVERY
STEP

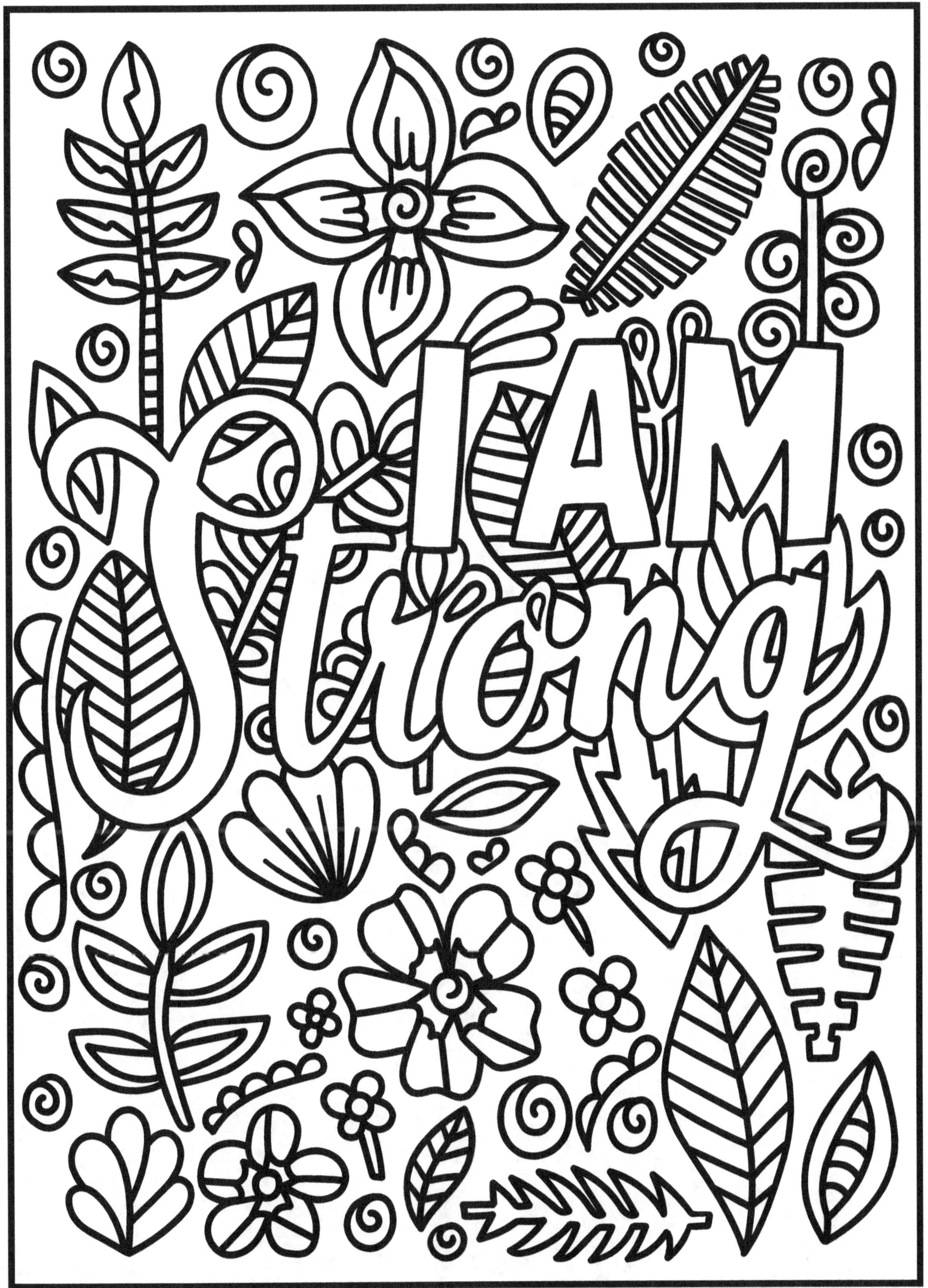

I AM
Strong

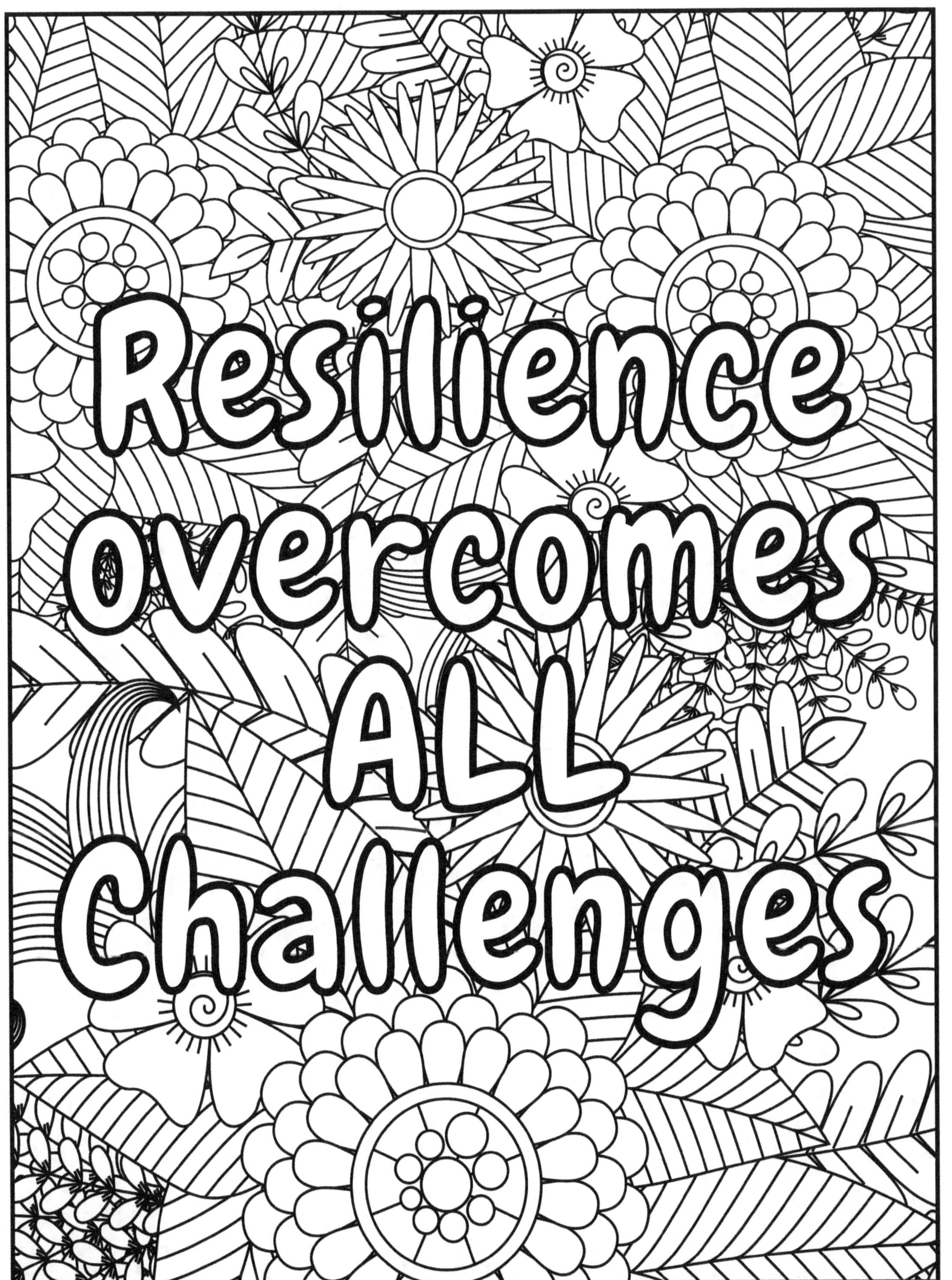

Resilience overcomes ALL Challenges

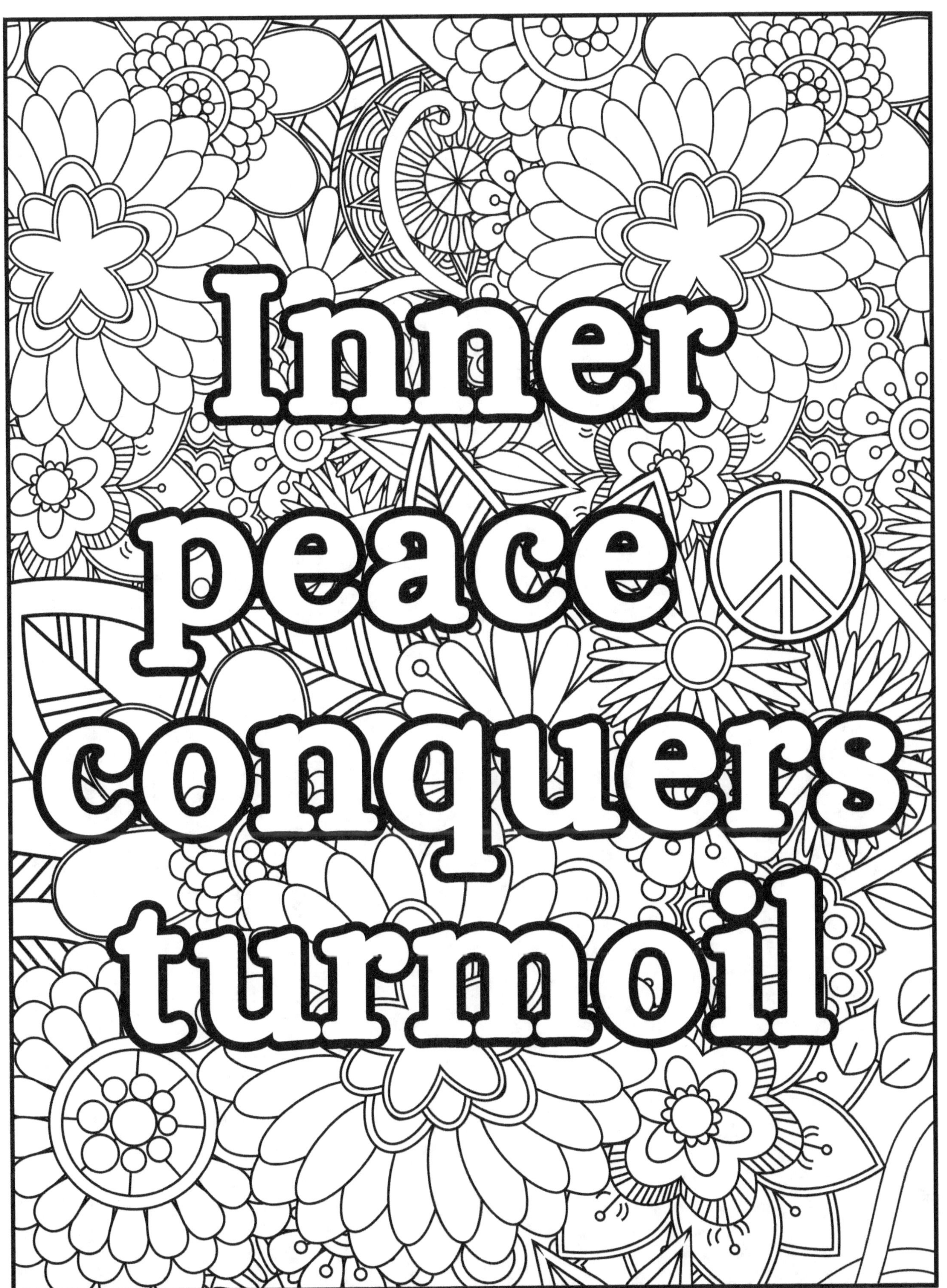

Inner
peace
conquers
turmoil

Strength

in every

Breath

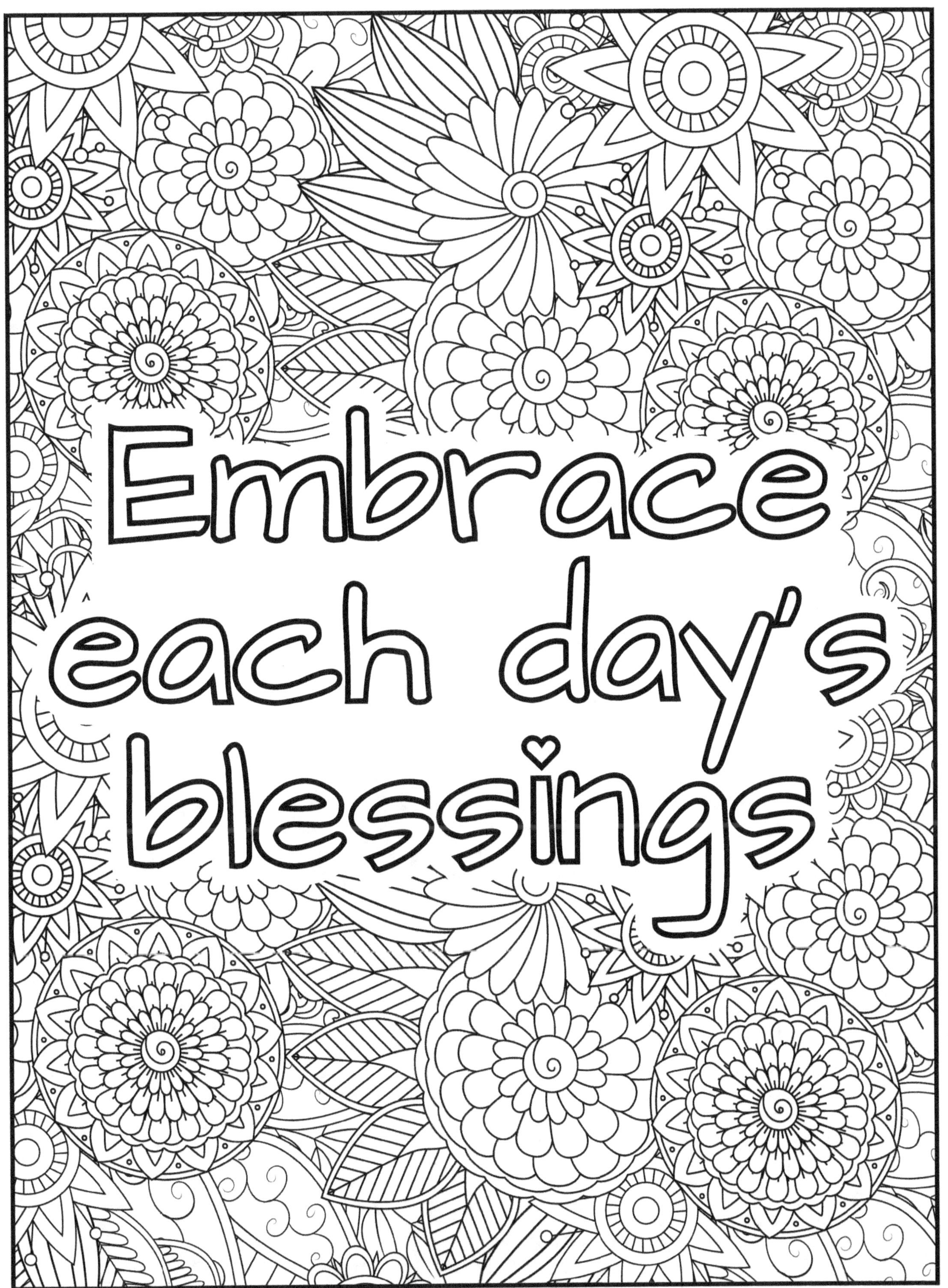
Embrace each day's blessings

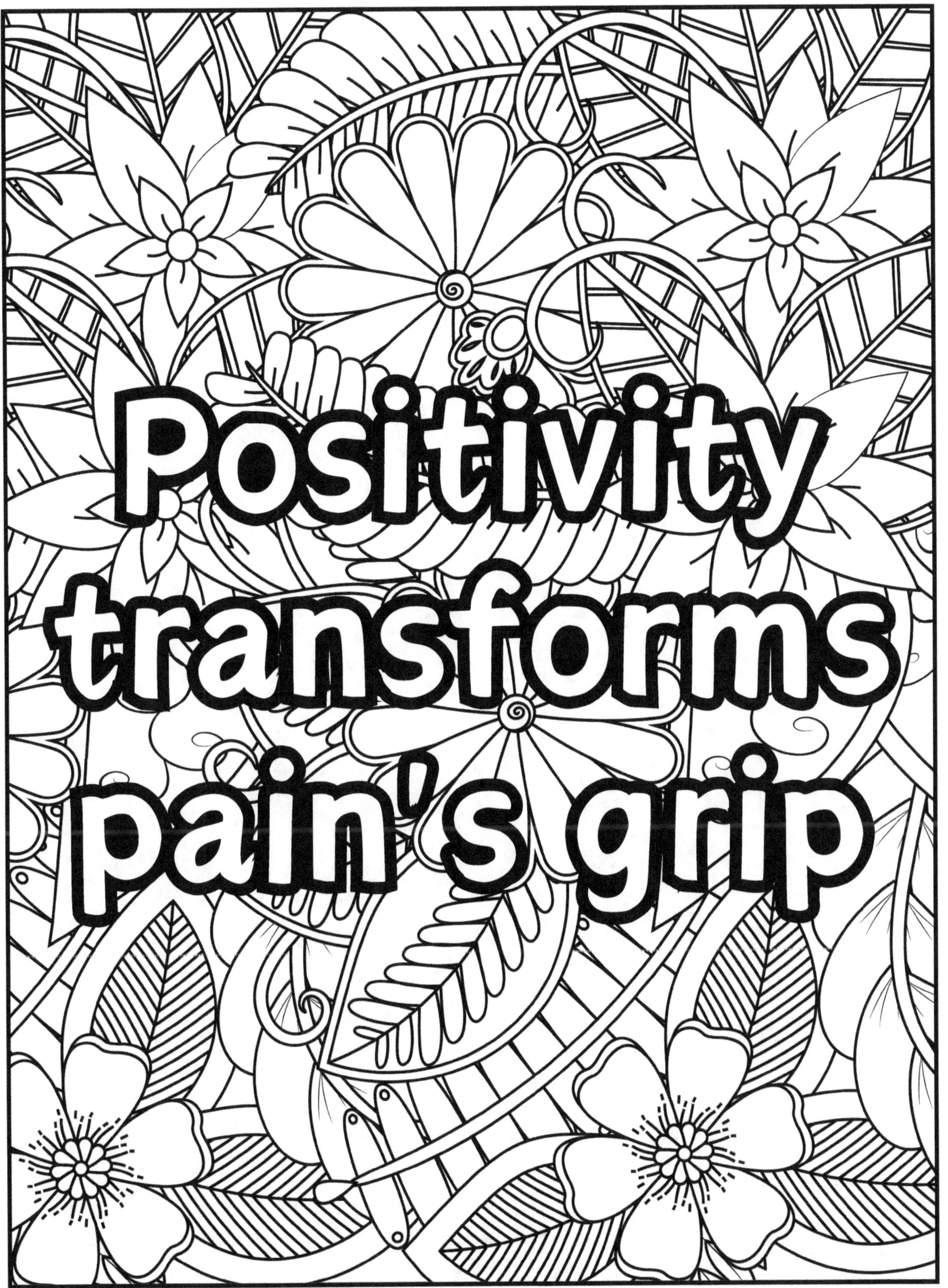

Positivity transforms pain's grip

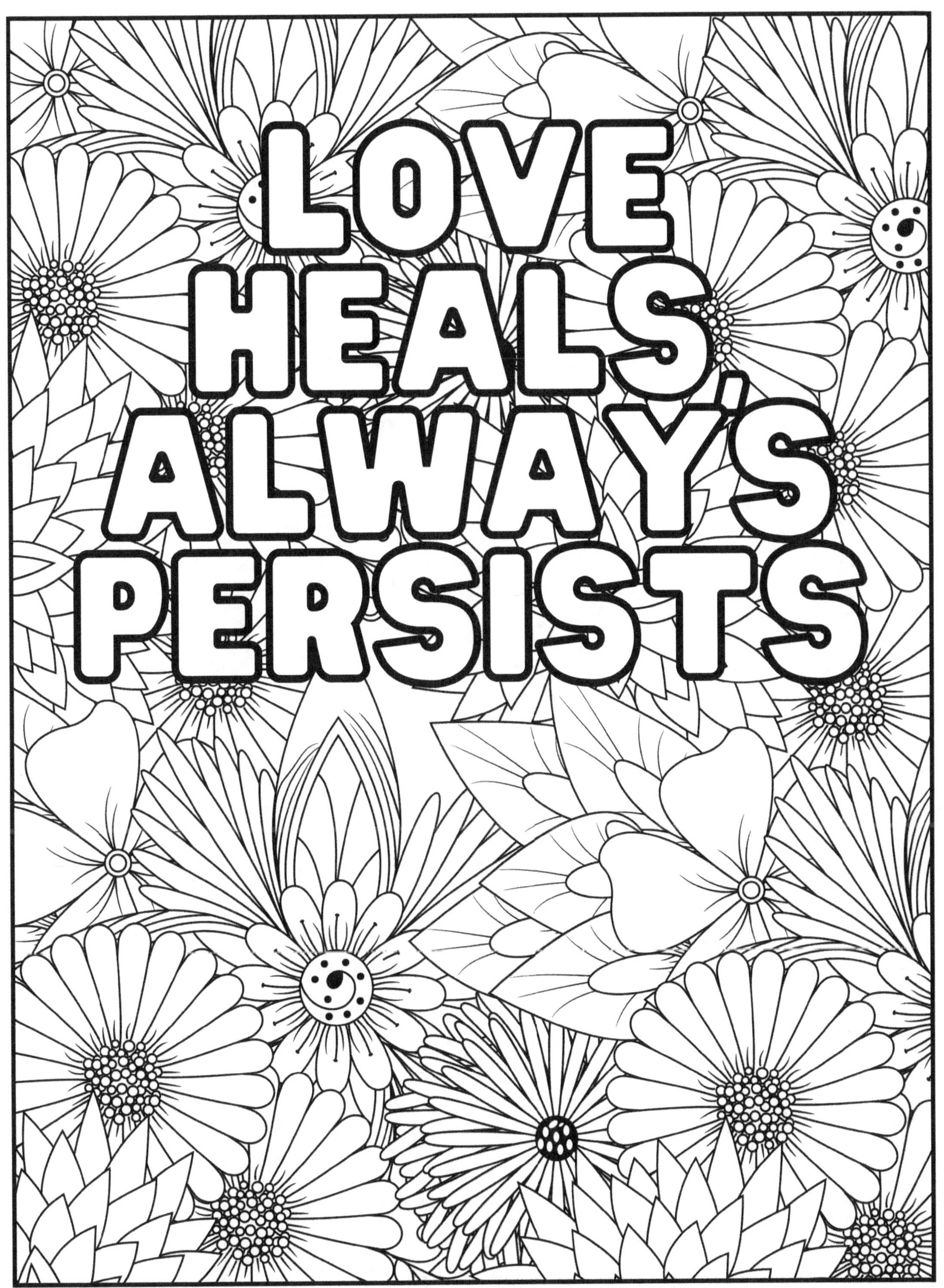

LOVE
HEALS,
ALWAY'S
PERSISTS

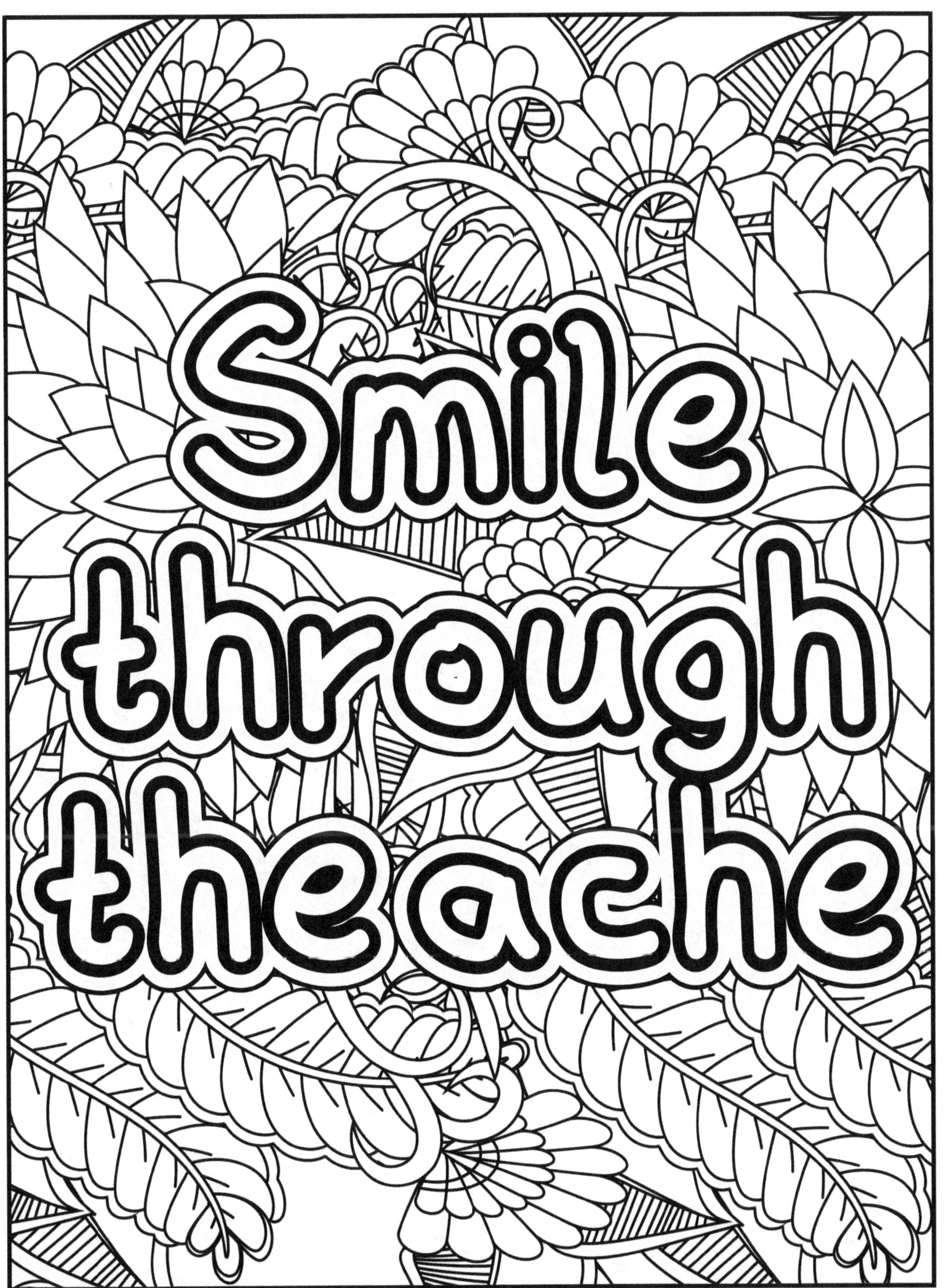

Smile
through
the ache

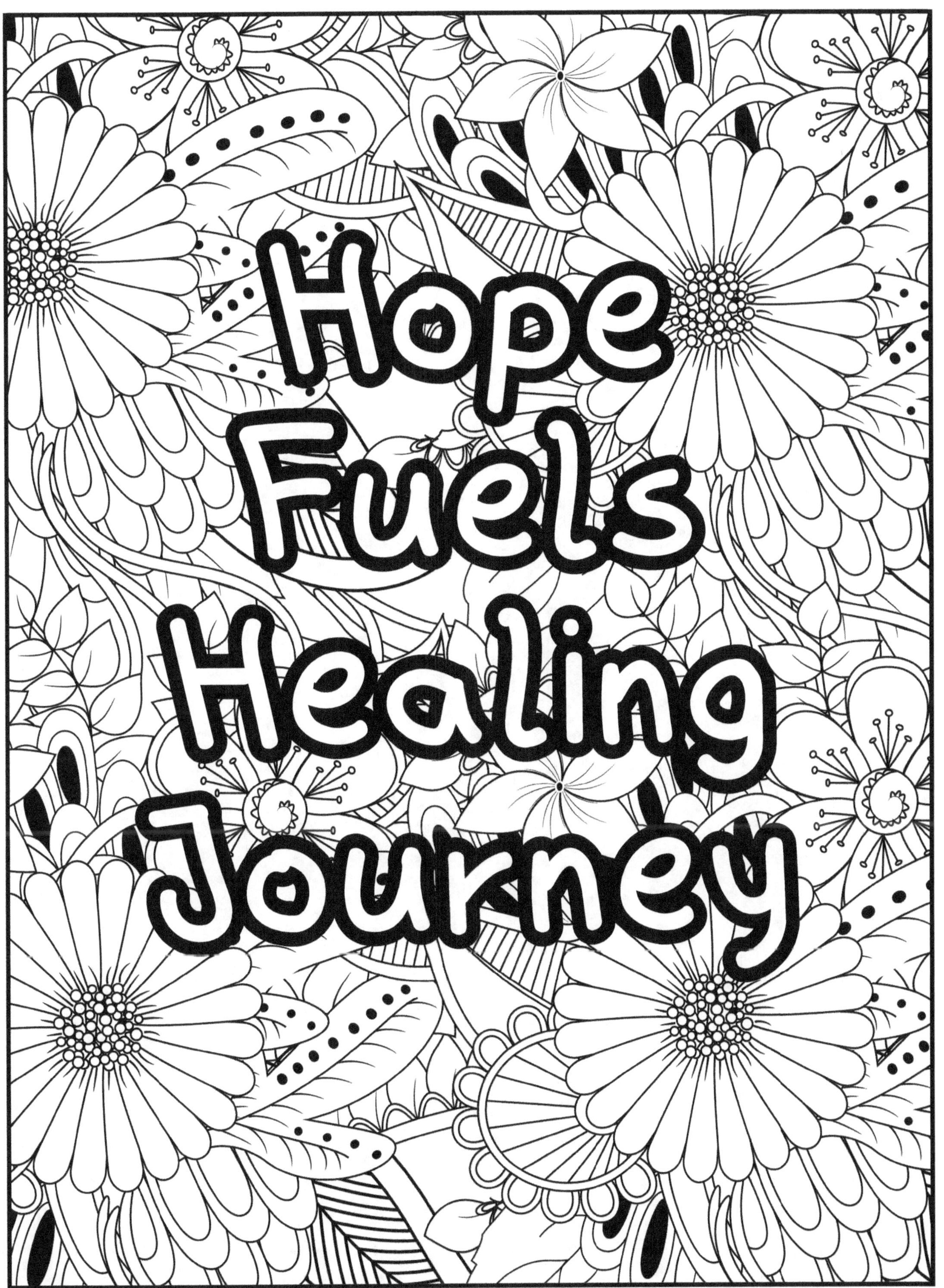

Hope
Fuels
Healing
Journey

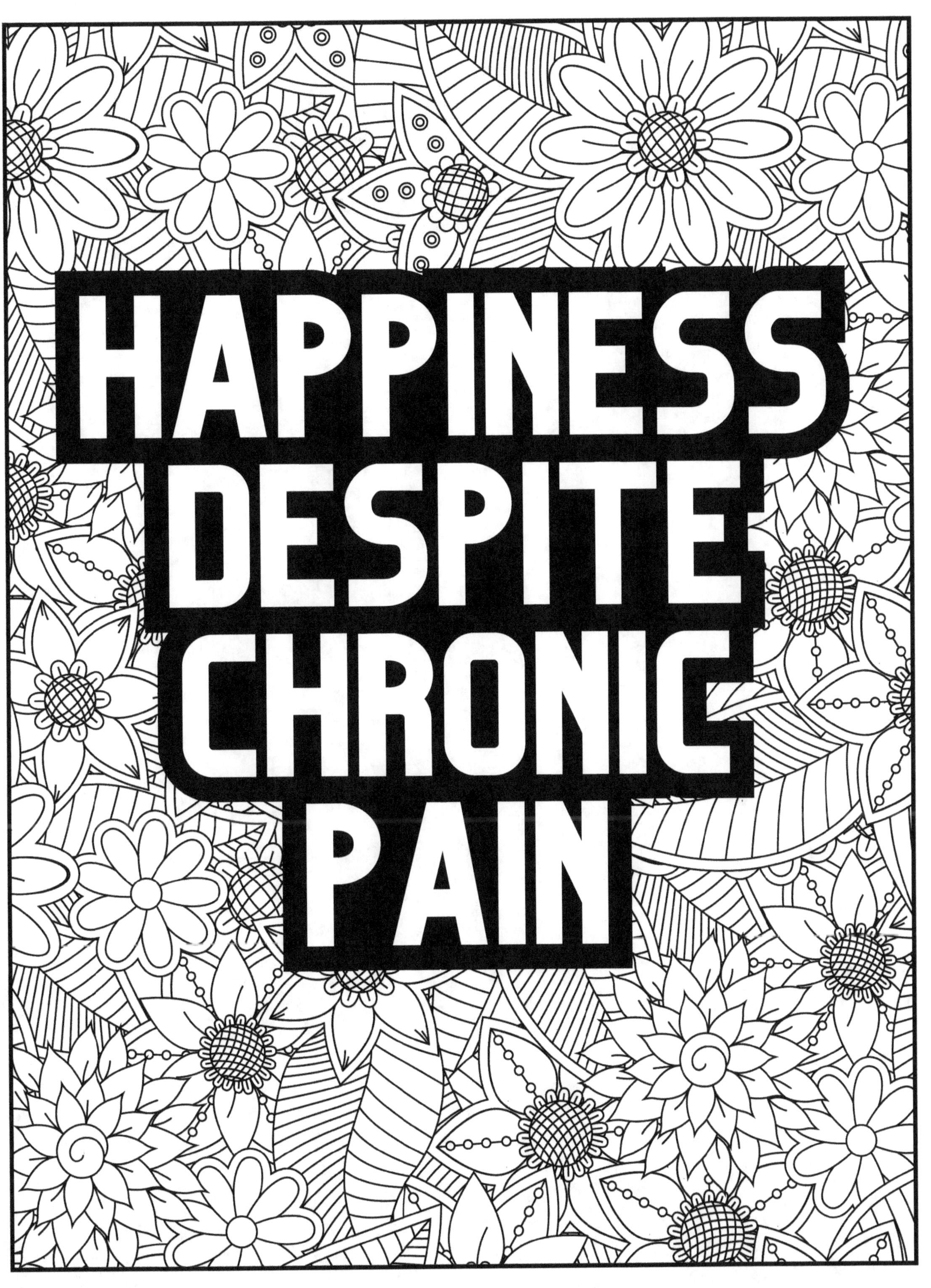

HAPPINESS
DESPITE
CHRONIC
PAIN

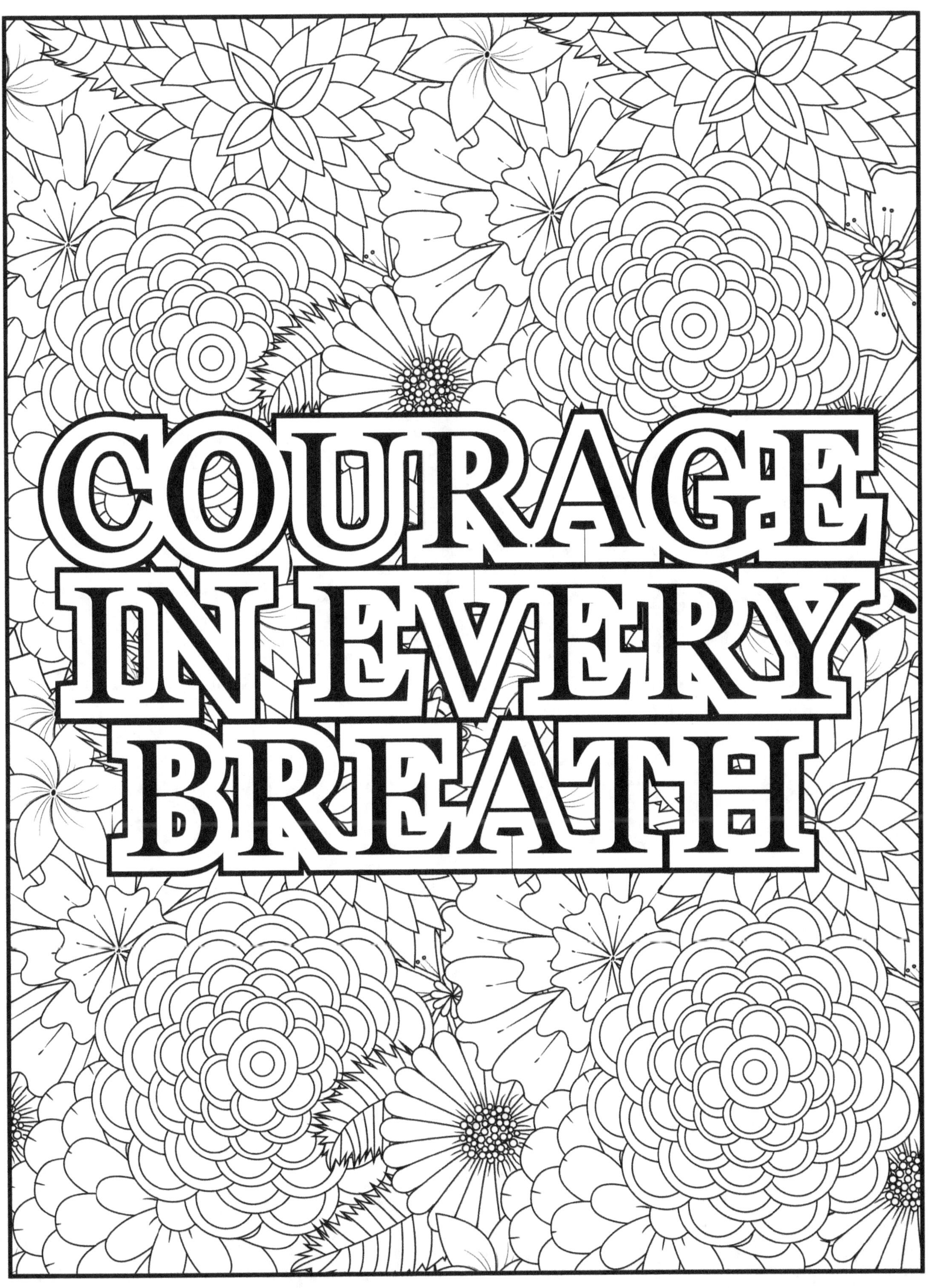

COURAGE
IN EVERY
BREATH

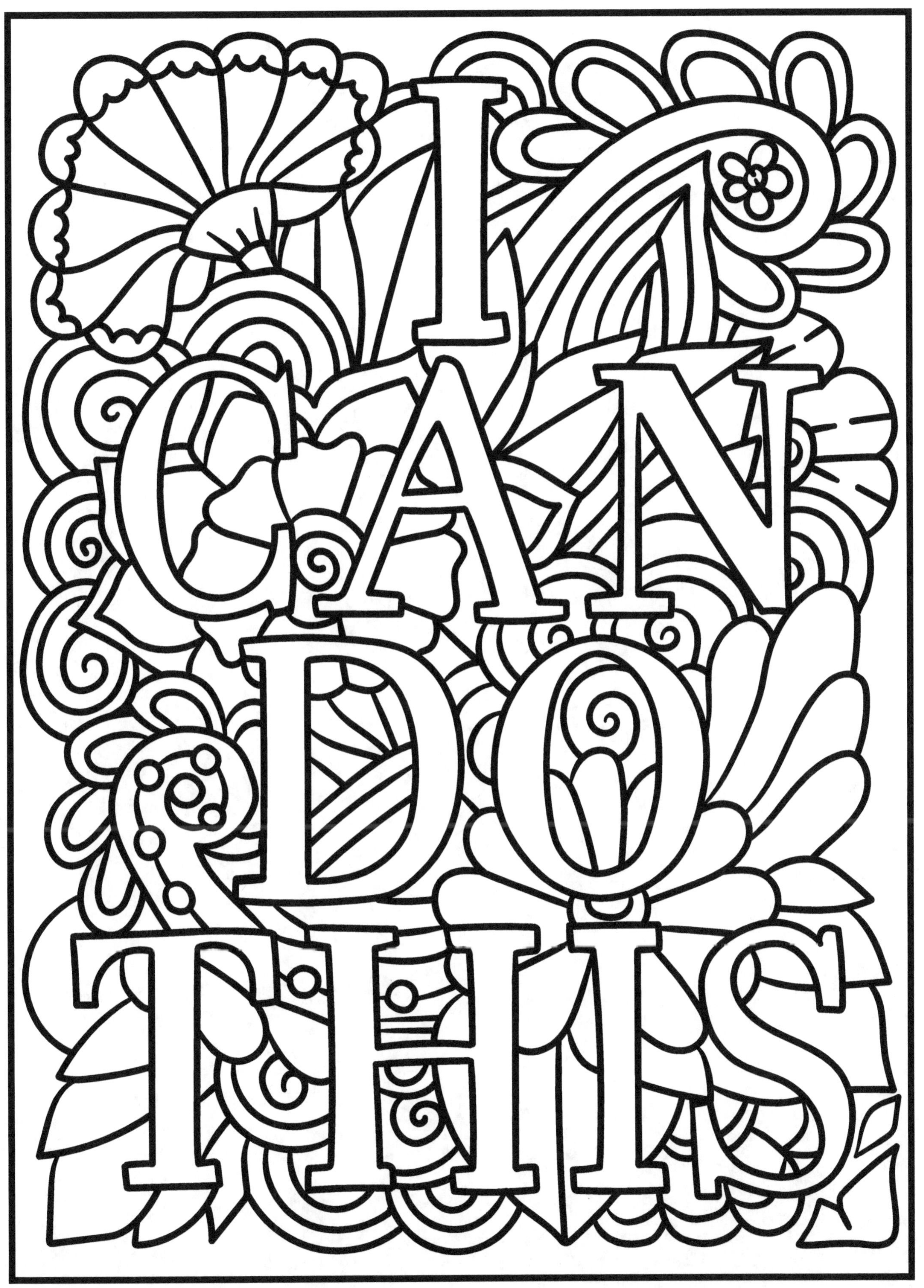

I CAN DO THIS

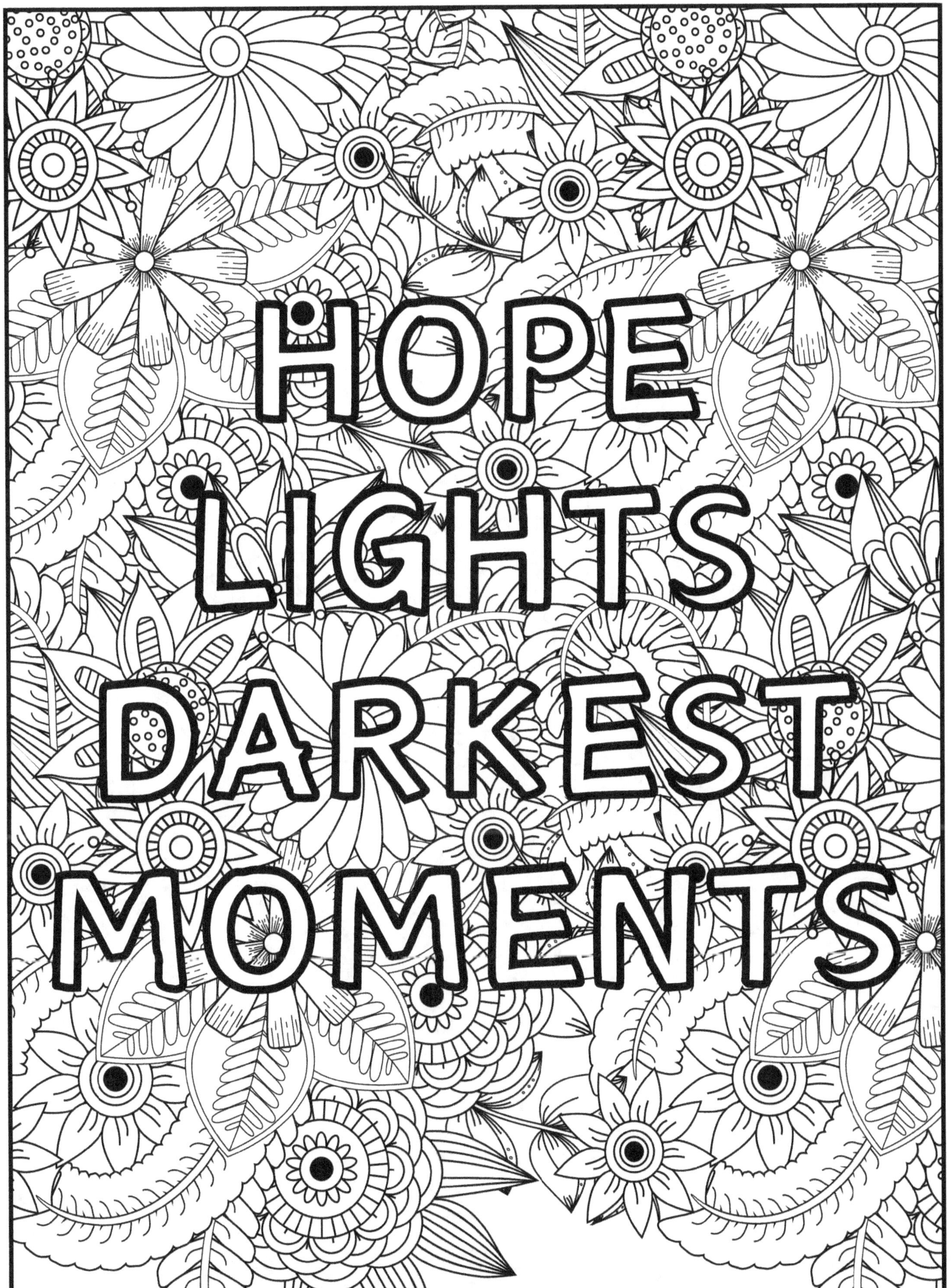

HOPE
LIGHTS
DARKEST
MOMENTS

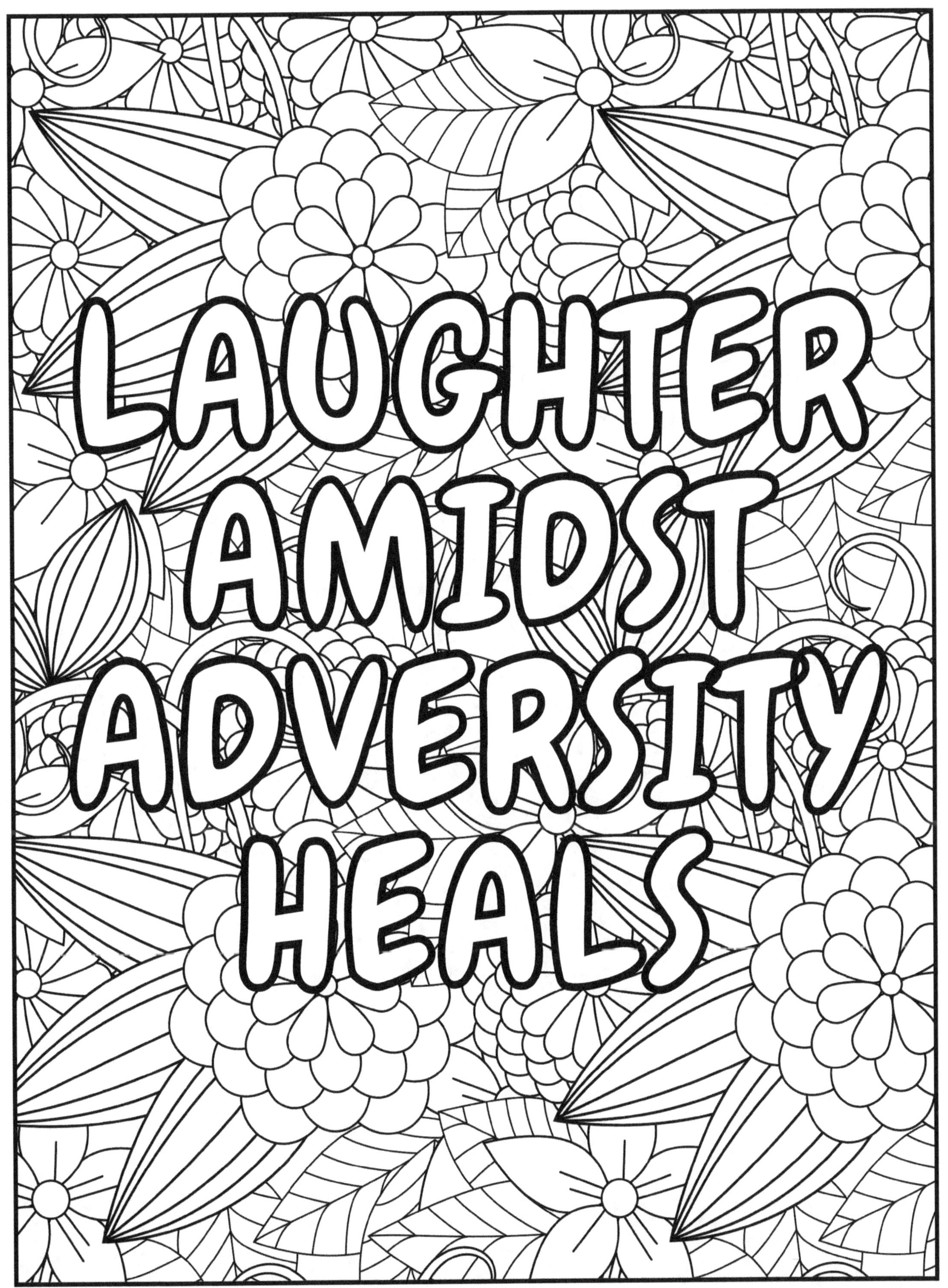

LAUGHTER
AMIDST
ADVERSITY
HEALS

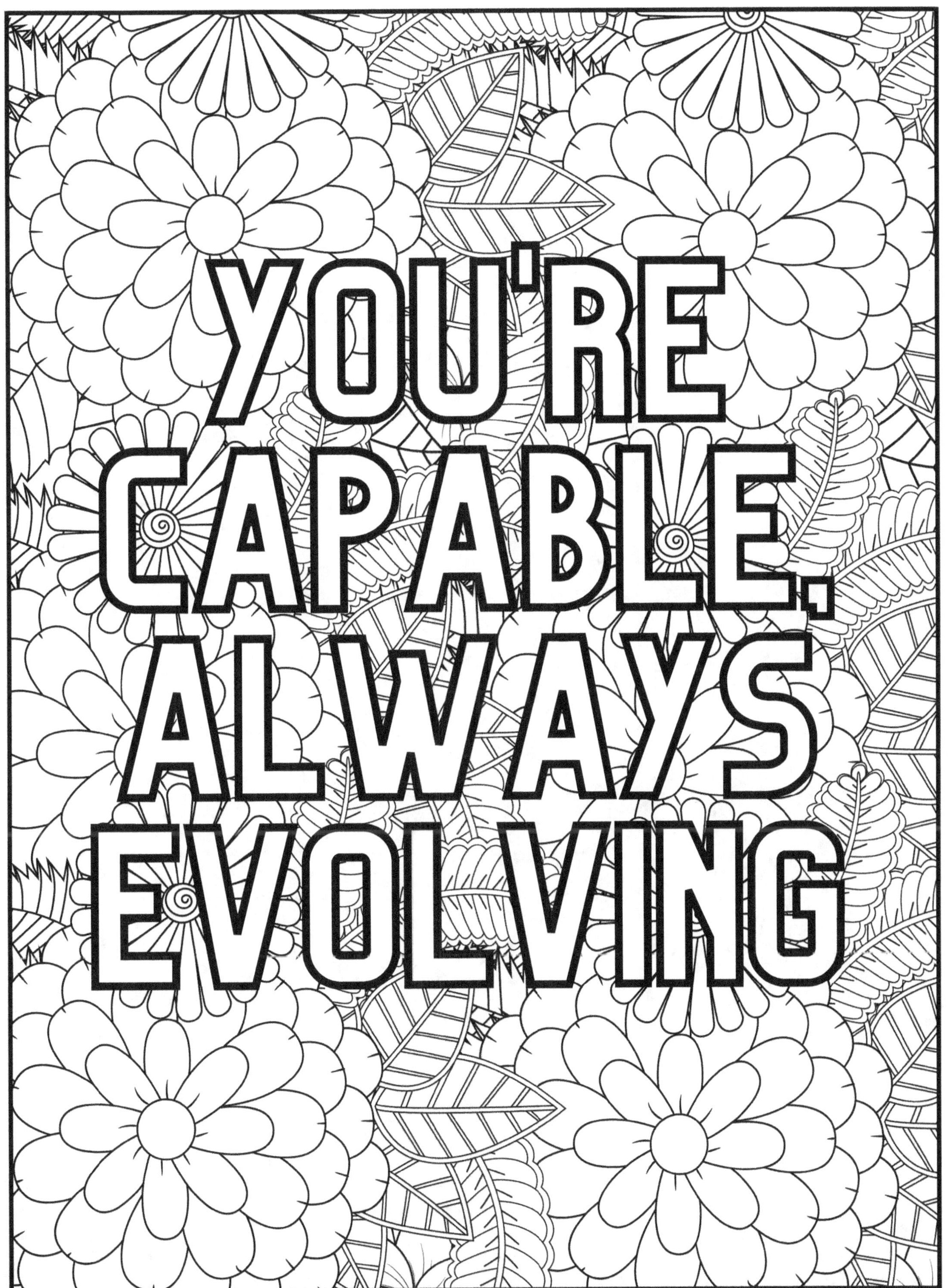

YOU'RE CAPABLE. ALWAYS EVOLVING

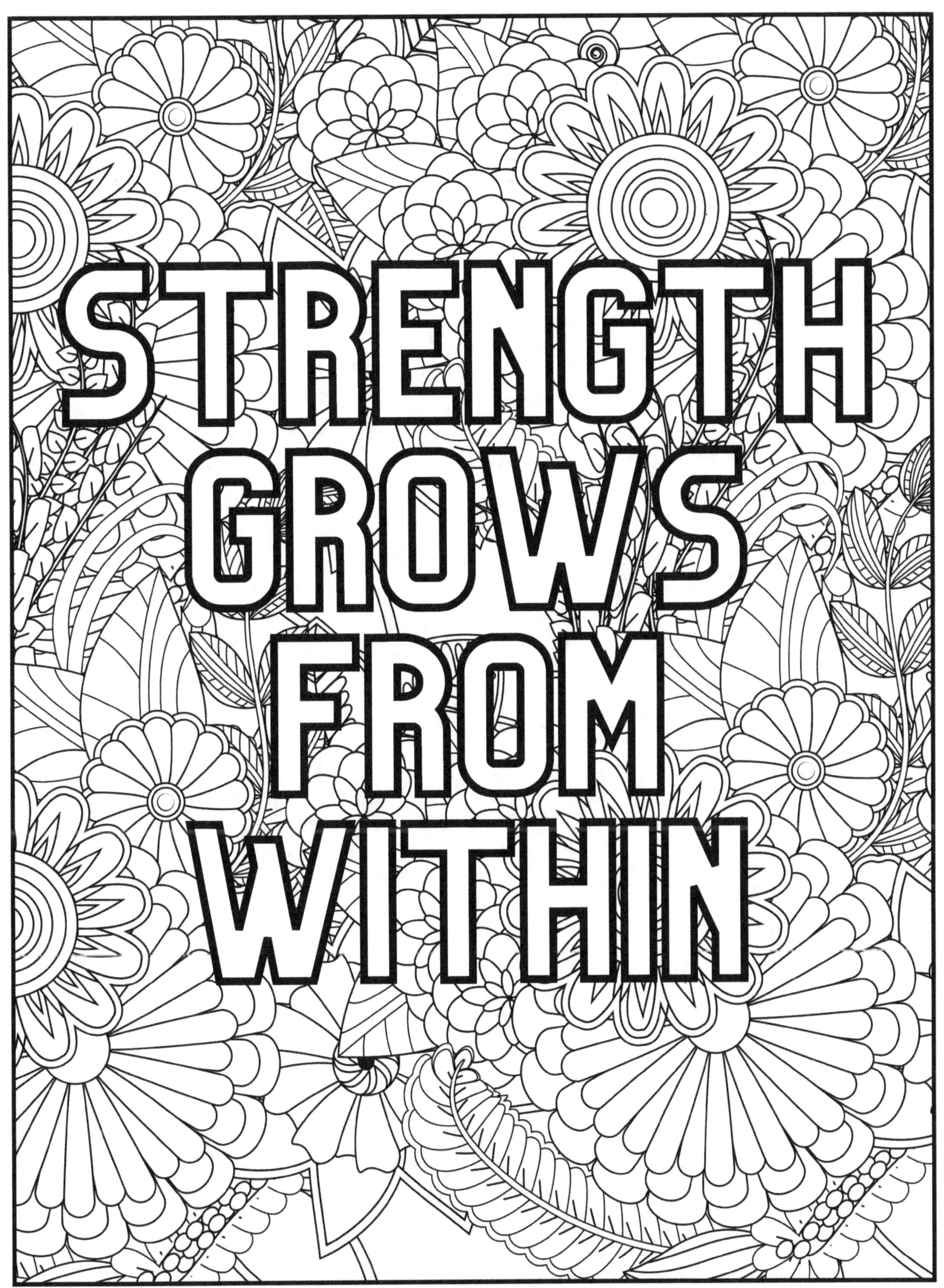

STRENGTH
GROWS
FROM
WITHIN

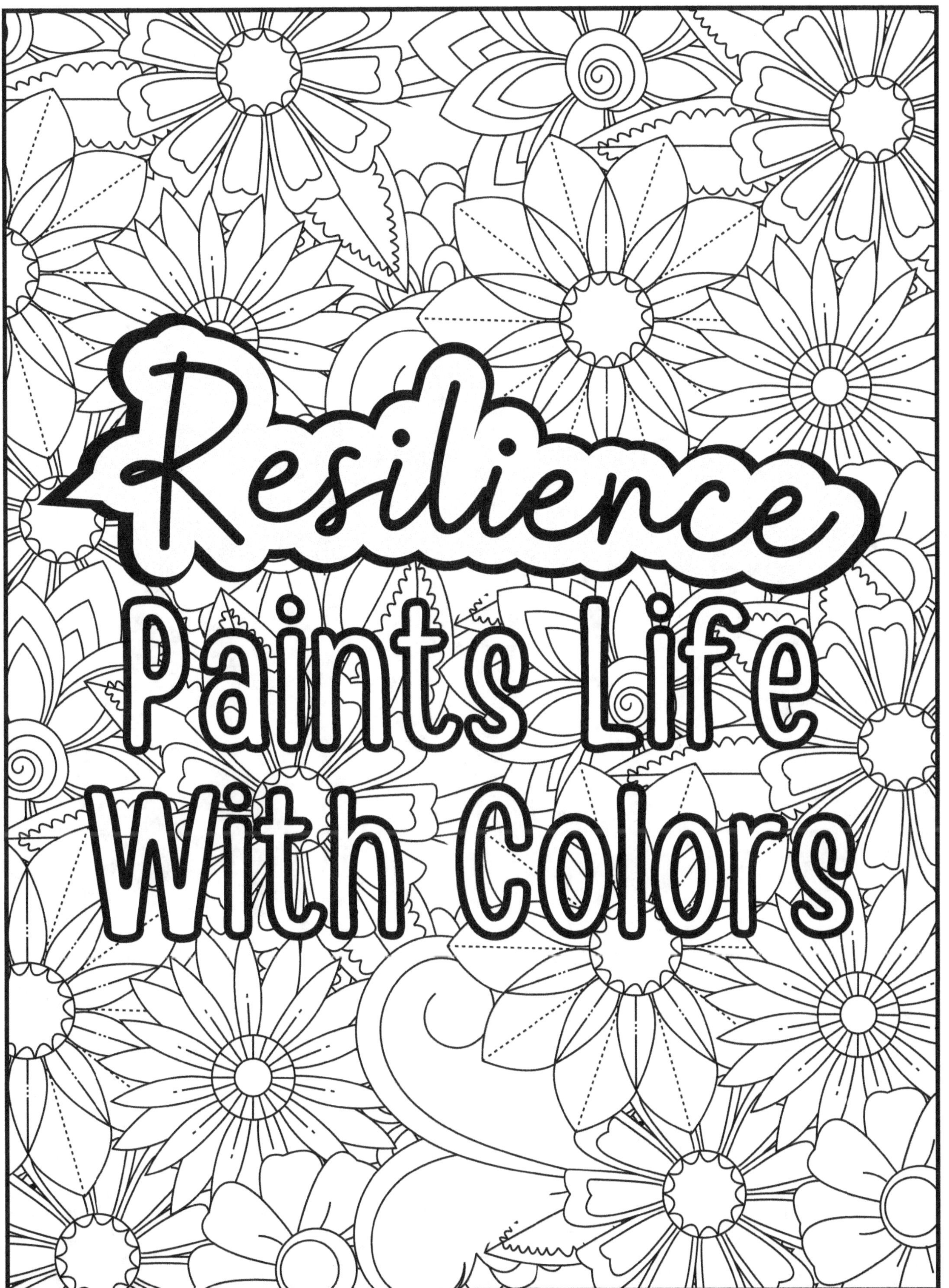

Resilience
Paints Life
With Colors

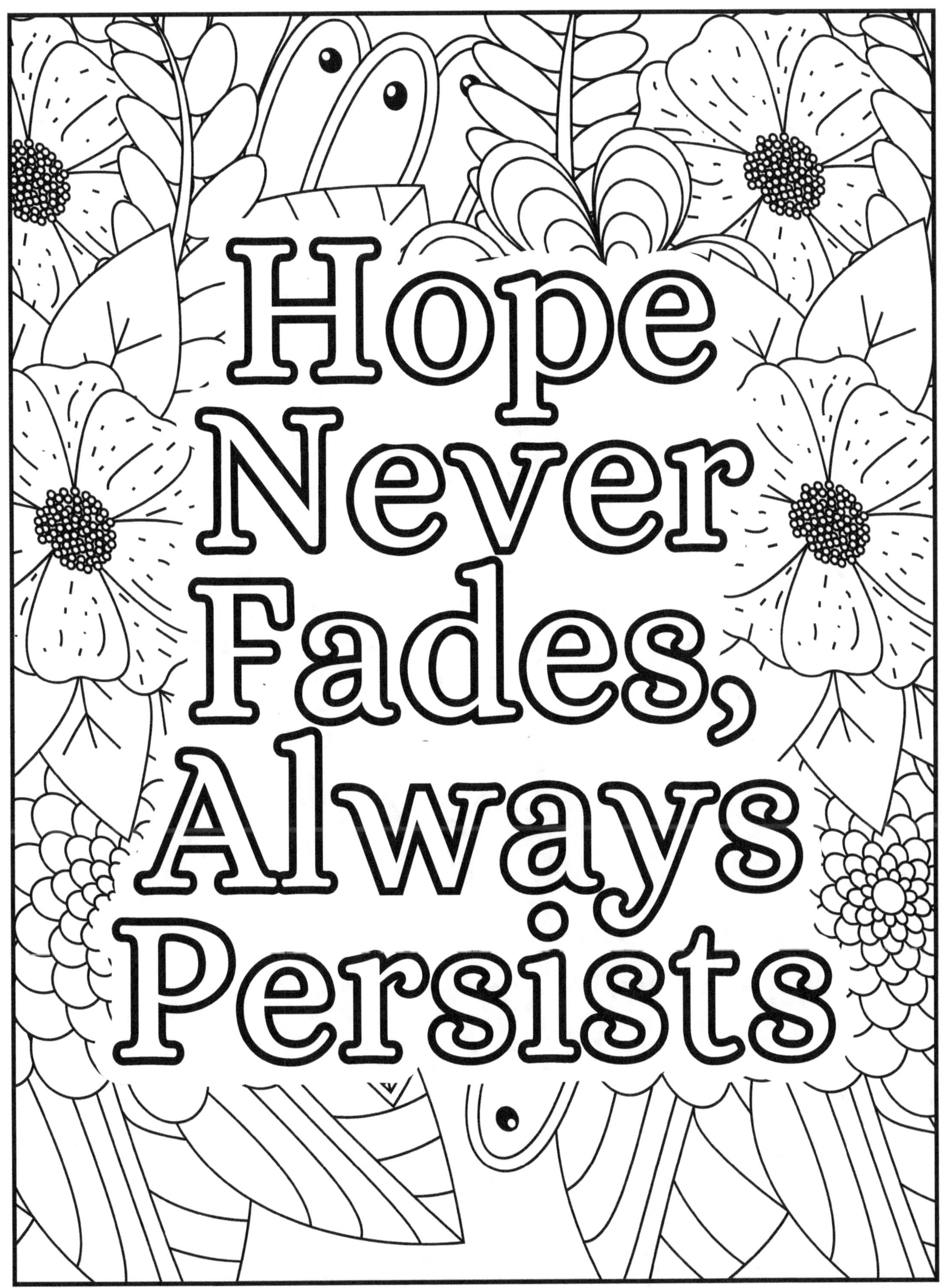

Hope
Never
Fades,
Always
Persists